PUBLISHER'S NOTE

The material in this book is selected from the book *Simplified "Taijiquan"* and from the pages of *CHINA SPORTS* magazine. Both published by the *CHINA SPORTS* Editorial Board, Beijing, China.

Traditional Chinese Fitness Exercises

Edited by
CHINA SPORTS
and
NEW WORLD PRESS

NEW WORLD PRESS
BEIJNG, CHINA

First Edition 1984

Second Printing 1995

ISBN 7-80005-310-5

Published by

NEW WORLD PRESS

24 Baiwanzhuang Road, Beijing 100037, China

Distributed by

CHINA INTERNATIONAL BOOK TRADING CORPORATION

35 Chegongzhuang Xilu, Beijing 100044, China

P. O. Box 399, Beijing, China

Printed in the People's Republic of China

CONTENTS

I. CHINESE FITNESS EXERCISES

A Historical Overview

(1)

Physical fitness exercises have been practised in China for thousands of years. The ancient Chinese were well aware of the importance of physical fitness and continuously sought ways for its improvement.

Through the Spring and Autumn and the Warring States Periods (770-221 B.C.), a method called *daoyin* was evolved for promoting health and curing certain diseases by combining regulated, controlled breathing with physical exercises. In a Western Han dynasty (206 B.C.-25 A.D.) tomb discovered several years ago on the outskirts of Changsha in Hunan Province, a silk scroll was found on which figures of *daoyin* exercises were drawn in different postures — sitting in meditation, stretching, bending, and squatting.

Towards the end of the Eastern Han dynasty (25-220 A.D.), the renowned medical scientist Hua Tuo (?-208) wrote: "The human body requires constant exercise", and "regular exercise aids digestion, stimulates circulation and helps the body to resist diseases". He created a set of exercises named *wuqinxi* (Five-Animal Play) mimicking the movements of the tiger, the deer, the bear, the ape and the bird. These exercises were then widely practised. Hua's disciple Fan A, a devotee of *wuqinxi,* was reputed to have lived to over 100. Wu Pu, another follower of Hua's, was said to have had sound teeth and acute hearing and sight when well into his 80s. Hua Tuo's inventive work had a far-reaching influence on the later development of physical exercises for improving health and for therapeutic purposes. During the Song (960-1279) and Ming (1368-1644) dynasties, there appeared a large number of exercise routines, including *baduanjin* (an eight-part exercise), *yijinjing* (a system of muscular exercise), *taijiquan* (traditional Chinese shadow boxing) and *qigong* (breathing exercises) which have retained their popularity up to this day.

(2)

Since the founding of the People's Republic in 1949, great efforts have been made to study and improve upon many traditional forms of fitness exercises in line with the policies of "making the past serve the present" and "weeding through the old to bring forth the new". In particular, the State Physical Culture and Sports Commission has organized specialists to conduct intensive research on *taijiquan,* the most popular of all traditional exercises. Their results have been compiled in a set of simplified *taijiquan* with 24 forms (see p. 38) and another more complicated set with 88 forms. Characterized by gentle, rhythmic movements, natural breathing and physical and mental coordination, *taijiquan* is of particular benefit to the old and the weak and those suffering from chronic diseases, though people of any age and at any fitness level can derive great benefits from practising it.

Qigong was cited for its therapeutic value in the *Huangdi Neijing* (*Yellow Emperor's Manual of Internal Medicine*), the oldest known Chinese medical treatise, which is believed to have been written in the Warring States Period. Intensive efforts are now being devoted to its study and application with rewarding results. Many new works have been written on the salubrious effects of *qigong* on the nervous, respiratory and digestive systems.

(3)

In recent years, many physical culture institutes, sanatoriums and hospitals in China have created a variety of remedial exercises by assimilating useful elements from traditional exercises. Based on modern theories of anatomy, sports physiology and biomechanics, these new exercises are designed to suit the needs of particular professions, such as steel-workers, coalminers and textile workers or to treat or prevent certain ailments, such as gastroptosis and eye strain. For example, at the Lake Taihu Workers' Sanatorium in Wuxi, Jiangsu Province, specialists have developed a set of lower back exercises derived from the traditional *wuqinxi*

(Five-Animal Play). These exercises produce results impossible to achieve by the use of drugs alone. Out of 109 cases under examination at the Lake Taihu Sanatorium, 89 showed cures or marked improvement after a year's practice of these ever effective exercises.

Daoyin Exercises

The silk scroll discovered in the Western Han tomb at Mawangdui near Changsha is covered with over 40 human figures in different postures outlined in black and painted in colour. Although some of the figures and explanatory Chinese characters are hardly distinguishable, after intensive research they have been identified as a series of daoyin diagrams. Judging from the figures' appearance and the descriptions of their movements, as well as the names of diseases referred to, they are the earliest extant depictions of exercises for promoting health and curing diseases.

It was on the bases of daoyin that Hua Tuo developed his wuqinxi exercises in the latter part of the Eastern Han dynasty. Books and diagrams about daoyin appeared in growing numbers in the Western Jin dynasty (265-317) and the time of the Sui and Tang dynasties (581-907), daoyin had evolved into other forms of fitness exercises, such as the popular baduanjin and taijiquan. Numerous illustrated books appeared dealing with these exercises in detail. Today these provide useful background information for the study of the daoyin paintings unearthed at Mawangdui.

These paintings depict men and women of different ages, dressed in various costumes and performing various movements, mostly bare-handed but occasionally with weapons. Traces of these movements can be found in warm-up exercises which became popular in later periods.

The *daoyin* exercises are beneficial for all the joints in the body and the shoulders, the waist, the knees and the respiratory organs. The methods of training and the principles involved are basically identical with those expounded in modern medical literature.

Figure 1. Bend and twist the body while grasping a pole.

Figure 2. Bend forward at the waist and touch the palms to the floor. Draw up the chin as much as possible.

Figure 3. Kneel on the floor and twist the trunk.

Figure 4. Sit on the floor with the knees drawn to the chest and clasp the knees with both hands.

Figure 5. Let both arms hang down naturally and bend the legs slightly at the knees.

Figure 6. Stand with the knees slightly bent and arms slightly extended.

The exercises for strengthening the muscles of the lower limbs and curing ailments in the knee joints, as shown in Figs. 5 and 6, are similar to those practised today. They testify to a thorough knowledge of the anatomy of the lower limbs and an elementary understanding of the laws of their movements.

In the case of upper limb movements, breathing

11

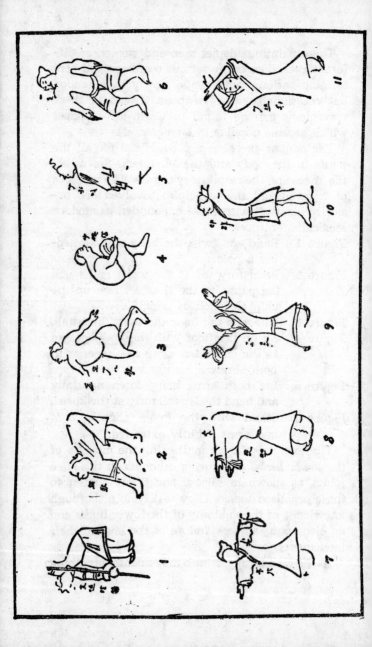

exercises go hand in hand with exercises of the shoulder joints to improve the functioning of the heart and lungs.

Figure 7. Stand erect and raise both arms out sideways from the body to shoulder height with the palms turned upward and chest expanded.

Figure 8. Stand erect, with both arms stretched forward at shoulder height and the palms facing downward.

Figure 9. Stand erect and raise both arms upward and outward like a bird spreading its wings.

Figure 10. Stand erect and raise both arms upward and backward while expanding the chest and breathing deeply.

Figure 11. Stand erect, raise both arms and cross them overhead.

With the help of modern medical knowledge, we can make scientific use of the *daoyin* movements and design setting-up or remedial exercises for various age groups of both sexes, as well as for strengthening different parts of the body.

Yijinjing

Yijinjing (limbering-up exercises for the tendons) is still used today as a means of keeping fit and as therapeutic exercise for orthopedic patients during convalescence. Just as the name implies — *Yi* (limber up or strengthen) + *Jin* (tendons) + *Jing* (method) — the exercises are designed to strengthen flaccid and frail muscles and tendons.

The movements of *yijinjing* are at once vigorous and gentle, and their performance calls for a unity of will and strength.

There are altogether 10 forms in this routine. Begin each form by looking straight ahead, clenching the teeth together tightly, opening the mouth slightly (or keeping it lightly closed) with the tongue resting on the hard palate. Do not exert force; do not throw out the chest or raise the shoulders; and stand up straight. Breathe naturally, remain relaxed, concentrate the attention on the navel, and swallow saliva when necessary. Be sure that each of these points is carried out throughout the entire exercise. These basics will not be repeated when each of forms is dealt with in detail below.

The main feature of this exercise is that all movements are executed with the palms. At the beginning, each movement can be repeated eight or nine times. After a period of training, the number may be gradually increased to 30 or more according to one's physical condition.

Form 1 Respiration with Fists Clenched

Starting Position:

Stand with feet shoulder-width apart. Clench both fists with the knuckles facing forward and the tips of both thumbs pressed lightly against the thighs (Fig. 1).

Method of Performing:

Use gentle abdominal respiration. When inhaling, distend the lower abdomen to the full; when exhaling, clench both fists tight. When inhaling

14

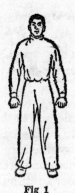
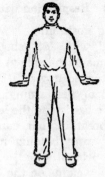

Fig 1   Fig 2

again, keep the fists clenched, and when exhaling, clench the fists more tightly than before. Repeat these movements.

Form 2   Respiration with Palms Pressing Downward

Starting Position:

Stand with feet shoulder-width apart. Press both palms downward with the fingers pointing sideways and the fingertips turned upward (Fig. 2).

Method of Performing:

The method of breathing in and out is the same as in Form 1; but when breathing out, press the palms downward with inner strength (do not bend the legs) with the whole body vibrating intensely. When inhaling, keep the body taut, and when exhaling again, press the palms downward with more force and raise the fingertips upward as much as possible, with the body vibrating still more intensely. Repeat these movements.

15

Form 3　Respiration with Palms Upward

Starting Position:

Stand with feet shoulder-width apart. Raise both arms to the side at shoulder height, with the palms turned upward (Fig. 3).

Method of Performing:

Inhale to distend the lower abdomen to the full. When breathing out, concentrate on the palms as if they were holding up heavy weights. Every time you breathe out, exert more inner strength as if the weights on the palms were getting heavier and heavier (maintain the position of the palms). Repeat these movements.

Form 4　Respiration with Palms Extended Outward

Starting Position:

Stand with feet shoulder-width apart. Raise both arms to the side at shoulder height, with the fingers pointing upward and the palms facing

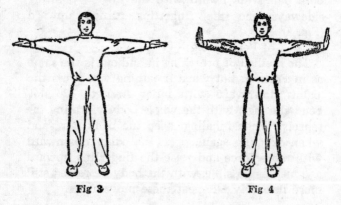

Fig 3   Fig 4

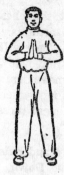

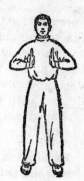

Fig 5a   Fig 5b

outward. Bend the fingertips towards the head as much as possible so that the palms extend outward (Fig. 4).

Method of Performing:

Method of breathing is the same as before. When exhaling, extend the palms outward with inner strength as if pushing something away, with the whole body vibrating intensely. Exert more force with each push so that you feel as if the palms were extending further and further outward. Repeat these movements.

Form 5   Open and Closed Respiration

Starting Position:

Stand with feet shoulder-width apart. Place the palms together in front of the chest, with the fingers turned upward and the tips of the thumbs pressed against the chest (Fig. 5a).

Method of Performing:

When breathing in, keep the elbows level and draw the palms slowly apart, with the thumbs pressed lightly against the chest, until they come to the sides of the armpits. Meanwhile the whole body vibrates intensely (Fig. 5b). When breathing out, the palms move slowly back to the starting position. The movements should be coordinated with the breathing, which should be slow, relaxed, and even. Repeat these movements.

Form 6 Respiration with One Hand Raised High and the Other Hanging Down

Starting Position:

Move the left foot a step to the left and bend the left leg at the knee, keeping the right leg fully extended. The body remains straight. Raise the left hand with the palm facing upward, while the right hand hangs naturally by the right side of the body with the fingertips pointing downward and the palm facing the thigh (Fig. 6a).

Method of Performing:

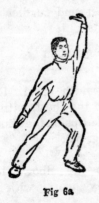 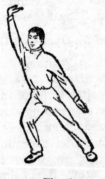

Fig 6a   Fig 6b

Throughout the breathing process, keep the position of the body unchanged. While breathing, extend both arms as fully as possible by exerting inner strength, and allow the whole body to vibrate intensely. Repeat these movements and relax naturally; then move the right foot a step to the right and do the exercises in this position (Fig. 6b).

Form 7 Respiration While Bending and Straightening

Starting Position:
Stand with feet about 40 cm apart.
Method of Performing:
Stretch the arms forward and raise them to shoulder level, with the arms bent slightly and the palms facing upward (Fig. 7a). Then turn the palms downward (Fig. 7b), at the same time squatting down slowly while keeping the trunk erect. While repeating these movements, the

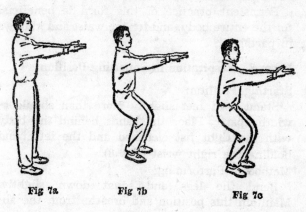

Fig 7a   Fig 7b   Fig 7c

19

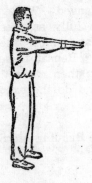

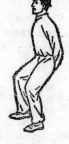

Fig 7d   Fig 8

degree of squatting may increase gradually until the thighs are parallel to the ground (Fig. 7c). Straighten up both legs slowly and turn the palms downward (Fig. 7d).

In this form, inhale when raising the hands and exhale when turning the palms downward and squatting. Repeat these movements.

Persistent practice of this form is beneficial for the entire body, and for the waist and kidneys in particular.

Form 8   Respiration in Squatting Position

Starting Position:

Stand with feet slightly more than shoulder-width apart. Place the hands behind the body with the right fist clenched and the left hand holding the right wrist (Fig. 8).

Method of Performing:

Bend the legs and squat down slightly. Maintain this position and breathe from the abdomen. When breathing in, distend the lower abdomen to the full; when breathing out, draw in the lower abdomen and contract the anus as if trying to hold back the stool. Repeat these movements.

This form is similar to a standing form in *qigong*. It is useful in treating neurasthenia, hypertension and other ailments. Constant practice will help strengthen the lower limbs.

Form 9 Respiration in Bending Position

Starting Position:

Stand with feet shoulder-width apart (Fig. 9a). Method of Performing:

Bend over slowly to an angle of 90 degrees, at the same time letting the hands hang down naturally (Fig. 9b). The shoulders should vibrate slightly as the hands continue to drop, with the palms turned inward and fingertips pointing downward. Do not exert any strength with the hands. Inhale when bending forward and exhale

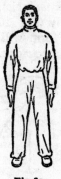

Fig 9a

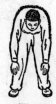

Fig 9b

when straightening up. Repeat these movements.

This form will help reduce excess fat in the abdomen and cure lumbago and backache.

Form 10 Respiration While Twisting the Body

Starting Position:

Stand at attention.

Method of Performing:

Move the left foot a step to the left. Twist the body to the left, placing the left hand on the lower back with the palm facing outward. Bend the right arm to form an arch and place it over the forehead, with the palm facing outward, about a fist's distance away from the forehead. Fix the vision on the right heel which remains on the ground (Fig. 10a). Stretch the waist as the body twists to the left; when breathing out, imagine that the centre of gravity is shifting to the right heel. Gradually twist the waist further around, and try to breathe from the abdomen (Fig. 10a).

Repeat the above movements, twisting to the right and the left alternatively (Fig. 10b).

Persistent practice of this form will help prevent and cure lumbago and backache.

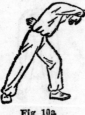

Fig 10a

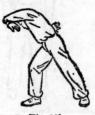

Fig 10b

Baduanjin: "Brocade" Exercises in Eight Forms

Baduan literally means "eight sections" and *jin*, "brocade". In the course of its development, *baduanjin* has appeared in a number of different versions. In the versions given below, Part I was devised by Zhong Li in the Tang dynasty (618-907) and rearranged by Li Shixin, a lecturer in the Physical Education Department of Beijing University. Part II was compiled by Zhuo Dahong, associate professor at Zhongshan Medical College, on the basis of several already existing versions.

(1)

Form 1 Holding Mt. Kunlun with Both Hands

Loosen your belt and clothing. Sit upright on a mat or towel with legs bent, the right calf over the left with both soles facing obliquely upward. Relax your whole body and concentrate your mind, looking straight ahead. Tap your teeth together lightly 36 times, with tip of tongue touching hard palate, and pause briefly. When your mouth becomes filled with saliva, swallow it in three gulps with a gurgling sound. Then cover your ears with your palms, fingers spread out like a fan. Place forefingers on middle fingers and tap on the back of the head 24 times. Take a deep breath, inhaling and exhaling slowly and evenly (Fig. 1).

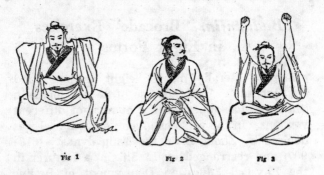

Fig 1   Fig 2   Fig 3

Form 2   Shaking the Heavenly Pillar

Sit upright with legs bent, right calf over the left, with soles facing obliquely upward. Place right palm on left above navel, with fingers slightly bent. Turn your head to the left, eyes looking backward as far as possible, for one or two seconds (Fig. 2). Then turn your head to the right, reversing the position of palms with a friction. Repeat 24 times. Keep torso erect while turning your head.

Form 3   Raising Arms

Sit upright with palms resting on bent knees, right calf over the left, both soles facing obliquely upward, and eyes straight ahead. Make relaxed fists and raise them overhead as if you were hanging from a horizontal bar (Fig. 3). Move your tongue around the inside of your mouth 36 times to produce saliva, and swallow this in three mouthfuls. Close your eyes and imagine that your heart is being warmed by a torch with the flames spreading gradually throughout the whole body. Return palms to knees.

24

Form 4 Rubbing Lower Back

Strip to waist and sit upright with legs bent, right calf over the left and soles facing obliquely upward.

Rub palms together until they are warm and place them on your sides with thumbs pointing forward and fingers pointing obliquely downward (Fig. 4). Rub hands up and down at least 36 times against both sides of spinal cord. Put on your garment and place left palm below navel, right palm on back of left hand. Breathe gently and imagine a flame in your heart spreading down to the region below the navel. You feel warm all over.

Form 5 Twisting the Torso to One Side

Sit as in Form 4 with right hand on hip and left palm on abdomen above navel, eyes looking straight ahead. Turn left shoulder forward and right shoulder backward, and then return to original position. Repeat 36 times, turning head together with shoulders (Fig. 5).

Form 6 Twisting the Torso to Both Sides

Sit as in Form 4.

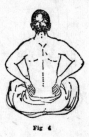

Fig. 4

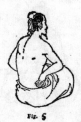

Fig. 5

25

Turn left shoulder forward and right shoulder backward, and then reverse this motion. Repeat 36 times, gradually increasing degree of rotation (Fig. 6). Place left palm on lower abdomen, and with right palm resting on back of left hand. Close your eyes gently and imagine a flame spreading from the lower abdomen up to the waist, then continuing up between the shoulder blades to the top of the head. Stretch legs forward, toes pointing up and muscles relaxed. Close your mouth lightly and take three deep breaths through your nose.

Form 7 Propping Up the Sky with Fingers Interlocked

Sit upright with legs bent, right calf over the left, both soles facing obliquely upward. With palms facing upwards, lock fingers together, pressing the little fingers against abdomen. Look straight ahead. Raise palms to chest level and then above head while gradually twisting wrists until palms face upward (Fig. 7). Then return

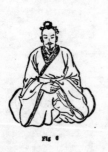

Fig 6

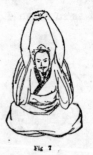

Fig 7

palms to abdomen. Repeat nine times, inhaling when raising palms and exhaling when lowering them.

Form 8 Pulling Toes with Both Hands

Sit upright with legs stretched forward, feet shoulder-width apart. Place palms on floor at your sides, with thumbs touching body and fingers pointing forward. Look straight ahead.

Bend forward and grasp the ball and toes of one foot with both hands, pulling back the top of the foot as you thrust heel forward. Repeat with the other foot. Eyes should follow the moving foot. Repeat 12 times, taking a deep breath each time (Fig. 8). Sit quietly for a few moments with eyes and mouth gently closed. Move your tongue around inside your mouth to produce saliva and swallow it quickly. Repeat six times. Then shrug your shoulders and twist your waist. Finally relax your whole body.

This set of exercises may be practised both in the morning and in the evening. Persistent practice will sharpen your appetite, help you to sleep more soundly and increase your resistance to disease.

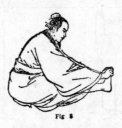

Fig 8

Form 1 Propping Up the Sky with Fingers Interlocked

Starting position: Stand at attention with heels together or feet separated slightly, with toes on floor and arches lifted. Arms hang naturally at your side. Place tip of tongue lightly against roof of the mouth and breathe through your nose. Look straight ahead and relax all joints. Maintain this stance for several minutes (Fig. 1).

Movements:

1. Raise arms slowly and interlock fingers overhead, palms turned up as if propping up the sky; raise heels at the same time (Fig. 2).

2. Return to starting position.

Repeat these movements many times. You may coordinate them with respiration, inhaling when raising arms and exhaling when lowering them.

This exercise helps to increase lung capacity

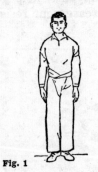

Fig. 1

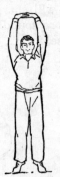

Fig. 2

and relieve fatigue. It also aids in strengthening the muscles and bones of the back.

This exercise prepares muscles and internal organs for the forms which follow.

Form 2 Drawing the Bow on Both Sides

Starting position: Stand at attention.
Movements:

1. Take a step to the side with the left foot and bend both legs. This is the "on horseback form". Cross arms at chest level, right arm on the outside. Extend left arm to the left with forefinger pointing upward, thumb stretched back, and other fingers bent. Turn head to the left and look at left forefinger. At the same time make a fist with the right hand and extend it to the right at shoulder level with arm bent as if you were drawing a bow (Fig. 3).

2. Return to starting position.

3. Repeat 1, reversing sides.

4. Return to starting position.

Repeat these movements many times. You may also coordinate them with respiration, inhaling when drawing arms sideways and exhaling when returning to starting position.

This exercise helps strengthen the muscles of the chest, arms and shoulders, and stimulate the respiratory and circulatory functions.

Form 3 Raising One Arm

Starting position: Stand at attention with heels together or feet shoulder-width apart, arms

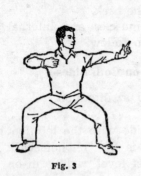

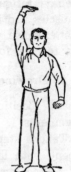

Fig. 3   Fig. 4

hanging naturally at both sides.

Movements:

1. Raise right hand overhead with palm up and fingers together pointing to the left. At the same time press left hand downward, with palm facing the floor and fingers pointing forward (Fig. 4).

2. Return to starting position.

3. Repeat 1, reversing sides.

4. Return to starting position.

Repeat these movements many times. You may coordinate them with respiration, inhaling when raising and lowering hands, and exhaling when returning to starting position.

This exercise stimulates the internal organs and aids in the prevention of gastro-intestinal disorders.

Form 4   Turning Head to Look over the Shoulder

Starting position: Stand at attention with palms pressed lightly against thighs.

Movements:

1. Turn head slowly to the left and look over left shoulder.

2. Return to starting position.

3. Turn head slowly to the right and look over right shoulder (Fig. 5).

4. Return to starting position.

Repeat these movements many times. You may coordinate them with respiration, inhaling when turning head and exhaling when returning to starting position.

This exercise aids in strengthening the muscles surrounding the eye sockets, strengthening the neck muscles to prevent cervico-vertebral ailments, and in stimulating blood circulation in the head to eliminate weariness, dizziness and other functional disturbances of the central nervous system. It is particularly beneficial to sufferers of hypertension and arteriosclerosis.

Form 5   Swaying Head and Buttocks

Starting position: Stand with feet about three

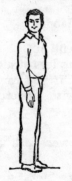

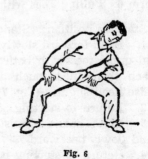

Fig. 5   Fig. 6

foot-lengths apart and bend knees to assume the "on horseback" form. Place palms on thighs with thumbs pointing backward.

Movements:

1. Lower head, bend trunk forward, and sway to the left side. At the same time, sway buttocks to the right, aiding the movement by stretching out left leg and hip. Hands may move along with trunk movement (Fig. 6).

2. Return to starting position.

3. Repeat 1, reversing sides.

4. Return to starting position.

Repeat these movements many times. You may coordinate them with respiration, inhaling when swaying trunk and exhaling when returning to starting position.

This exercise aids in "ridding the heart of fire", a traditional Chinese medical term which means overcoming strain in the nervous system caused by physical exertion and which cannot be eased through rest.

Form 6 Pulling Toes with Both Hands

Starting position: Stand at attention.

1. Bend forward slowly, keeping legs straight, and grasp toes with both hands. If you cannot reach them, just touch ankles with fingertips. Raise head slightly (Fig. 7).

2. Return to starting position.

3. Place hands against the lower back and bend slowly backward.

4. Return to starting position.

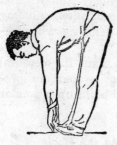

Fig. 7

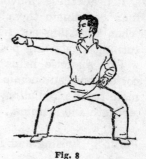

Fig. 8

Repeat these movements many times. Breathe as naturally as possible.

This is an exercise for the waist which aids in developing the lumbar muscles and preventing and curing strains. It is also effective in improving the functions of kidneys and the adrenal glands. People suffering from hypertension and arteriosclerosis should not lower head too much when doing this exercise.

Form 7   Clenching Fists and Looking with Eyes Wide Open

Starting position: Assume the "on horseback" position, with toes gripping the floor, hands tightly clenched at the waist, and knuckles facing down. Look ahead with eyes wide open (Fig. 8).

Movements:

1. Thrust right hand slowly to the right until arm is fully extended, with knuckles facing up.
2. Return to starting position.
3. Repeat 1, reversing sides.
4. Return to starting position.

33

Repeat these movements many times. You may coordinate them with respiration, inhaling when thrusting out fist and exhaling when returning to starting position.

This exercise helps to stimulate the cerebral cortex and autonomic nervous system, to promote blood circulation, and to build up muscular strength and stamina.

Form 8   Raising and Lowering the Heels

Starting position: Stand at attention, with palms pressed against the front part of thighs and legs straight.

Movements:

1. Raise both heels simultaneously, drawing head up as if there were a weight on its top.

2. Return to starting position.

Repeat these movements many times. You may coordinate them with respiration, inhaling when raising heels and exhaling when lowering them.

This exercise sets off light vibrations in the body which serve as finishing touches to the whole set of exercises.

Points to Remember

1. Exercise persistently. You'll never keep fit or cure chronic diseases if you "go fishing for three days and dry the net for two", as a Chinese saying goes.

2. When doing the exercises, relax both physically and mentally. When exertion is call-

ed for, use force gently by "integrating hardness with softness" — a principle governing all traditional Chinese fitness exercises.

3. Once you have relaxed, concentrate your attention on the acupuncture point of *dantian* (about 4 cm below the navel). Such concentration will aid abdominal respiration, promote blood circulation in the abdominal cavity and conduct *qi* (vital energy) to the lower part of the body.

4. Take a few deep breaths before you start the exercises. Breathe naturally and evenly. Practise in a place where the air is fresh.

5. Do not exercise within an hour after eating.

6. The duration of practice sessions and the intensity of exercise will vary from person to person. Generally speaking, you may stop when you start sweating lightly. In addition to *baduanjin*, you may take up other fitness exercises which suit your health condition, such as jogging, swimming, cold baths or sun baths.

II. TAIJIQUAN

Taijiquan

Though legends tell that some eight centuries ago, Emperor Xuanwu taught the art of *taijiquan* to an alchemist hermit in a dream, the available historical data seem to indicate that *taijiquan* was first devised in Henan Province some 300 years ago, in the late Ming and early Qing dynasties. In subsequent years foreign invasions and domestic peasant uprisings stimulated the diffusion of martial arts among the people, and a new form of boxing evolved. While earlier boxing styles emphasized quick movements and strong, vigorous punches, this new style followed the principles of "subduing the vigorous by the soft", "adapting oneself to the style of others" and "overcoming a force of 1,000 pounds with a force of four ounces".

In the past century, *taijiquan* has undergone significant changes, with its movements becoming more relaxed and graceful. Many moves requiring explosive strength disappeared, as did excessive foot stamping. Eventually *taijiquan* became popular with men and women, young and old alike, and increasing attention was paid to its hygienic and therapeutic value.

In the process of its development, *taijiquan* gradually evolved into many different styles, which need not be described here.

There were, however, five main schools, and numerous subdivisions under each school. Although each of the five has its own characteristic features, they share the following essentials:

First, the posture is natural and relaxed. Motion remains even and fluid, with the muscles neither stiff nor rigid. Breathing should be deep and regular. The practice of *taijiquan* requires a combination of vigour and gentleness — neither inertness nor rigidity is allowed.

Secondly, the mind should be tranquil but alert, with consciousness commanding the body, in order to achieve stillness within movement — a unity of stillness and motion.

Thirdly, body movements are well coordinated throughout the entire exercise period. Though the movements are gentle and slow, each part of the body is in constant motion. While practising *taijiquan*, the weight of the body is mainly borne by the waist and legs. A characteristic feature of *taijiquan* is that all movements are carried out in a half squatting position.

In 1956, a simplified set of *taijiquan* exercises based on the most popular sequences of the Yang school was issued. This series consists of 24 forms which progress logically from the easy to the difficult, and which take five minutes to complete. "Simplified *Taijiquan*" has proved to be a great stimulus to the popularization of the sport both in China and abroad.

Simplified *Taijiquan*

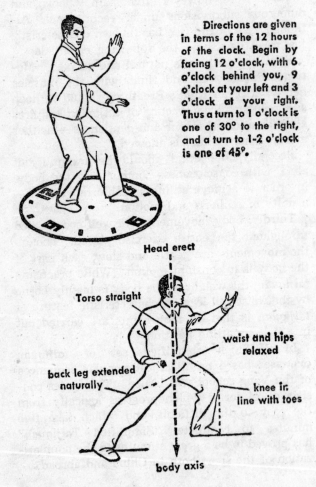

Directions are given in terms of the 12 hours of the clock. Begin by facing 12 o'clock, with 6 o'clock behind you, 9 o'clock at your left and 3 o'clock at your right. Thus a turn to 1 o'clock is one of 30° to the right, and a turn to 1-2 o'clock is one of 45°.

Head erect

Torso straight

waist and hips relaxed

back leg extended naturally

knee in line with toes

body axis

Series I
Form 1   Commencing Form

1) Stand naturally with feet shoulder-width apart, toes pointing forward, arms hanging naturally and hands at your sides. Look forward. (Fig. 1)

Points to remember: Hold head and neck erect, with chin drawn slightly inward. Do not protrude chest or draw abdomen in. Be relaxed but alert.

2) Raise arms slowly forward and upward to shoulder level with palms facing downward. (Figs. 2-3)

3) Keeping torso erect, bend knees while pressing palms down gently, with elbows dropping towards knees. Look forward. (Fig. 4)

Points to remember: Hold shoulders and elbows down. Fingers are slightly bent. Weight is equally distributed between both legs. While bending knees, keep waist loose and relaxed and buttocks slightly pulled in. The lowering of arms should coordinate with the bending of knees.

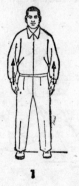 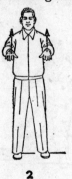 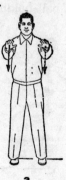

1   **2**   **3**

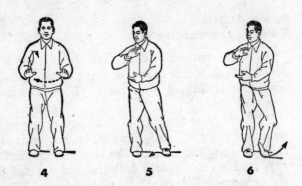

4　　　**5**　　　**6**

Series I
Form 2　Part the Wild Horse's Mane on Both Sides

1) Turn torso slightly to the right (1 o'clock) and shift weight onto right leg. Raise right hand until forearm comes in front of right part of chest, while left hand moves in a downward arc until it comes under right hand, palms facing each other as if holding a ball (henceforth referred to as the "ball-holding gesture"). Bring left foot next to

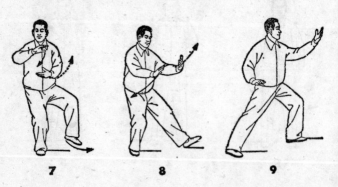

7　　　**8**　　　**9**

the right foot and rest toes on floor. Look at right hand. (Figs. 5-6)

2) Turn body to the left (10 o'clock) while left foot steps forward towards 8-9 o'clock, bending knee and shifting weight onto left leg, and right leg straightens with heel pressing down on floor to form a left "bow step". As you turn your body slightly leftward, gradually raise left forearm obliquely to eye level with palm facing obliquely upward and elbow slightly bent, and lower right hand beside right hip with palm facing downward and fingers pointing forward. Look at left hand. (Figs. 7-9)

3) "Sit back" slowly — move torso backward as if ready to take a seat — and shift weight onto right leg. Raise toes of left foot slightly and turn them outward before placing the foot flat on floor. Then bend left leg and turn body to the left (5 o'clock), shifting weight back again onto left leg. Make a ball-holding gesture in front of left part of chest, left hand on top. Then draw right foot

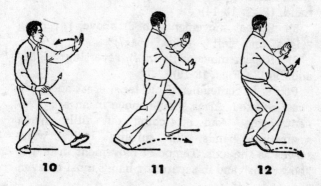

10   11   12

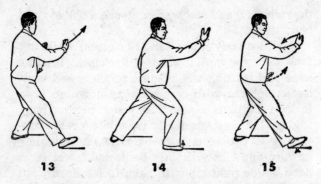

13 **14** **15**

forward to side of left foot and rest toes on floor.
Look at left hand. (Figs. 10-12)

4) Take a right bow step by moving right foot
a step towards 9-10 o'clock, straightening left leg
with heel pressing on floor and bending right leg
at knee. At the same time, turn body to the right
(8 o'clock), gradually raise right hand obliquely
upward to eye level with palm facing obliquely
upward and elbows slightly bent, and press left
hand down beside left hip with palm facing downward and fingers pointing forward. Look at right
hand. (Figs. 13-14)

5) Repeat movements in 3) above, reversing
"right" and "left". (Figs. 15-17)

6) Repeat movements in 4), reversing "right"
and "left". (Figs. 18-19)

Points to remember: Hold torso erect and keep
chest relaxed. Arms should move in an arc. Prevent arms from stretching out fully when
separating hands. In turning body, waist
serves as the axis. Tempo of movement in taking
"bow steps" and in separating hands must be even

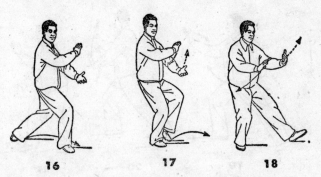

16   **17**   **18**

and synchronized. When stepping forward, place your foot slowly in position, heel coming down first. Knee of leg in front should not go beyond toes, which should point forward; the rear leg should be slightly straightened, forming an angle of 45 degrees with ground. Heels should not be in a straight line, the distance between them being 10-30 cm. Face 9 o'clock in the final position.

Series I
Form 3   The White Crane Spreads Its Wings

1) Turn torso slightly to the left (8 o'clock). Make a ball-holding gesture in front of left part of chest, left hand on top. Look at left hand. (Fig. 20)

2) Draw right foot a half-step towards left foot and then "sit back". Turn torso slightly to the right (10 o'clock). Look at right hand with weight on right leg, move left foot slightly forward and rest toes lightly on floor. (You have now taken a left "empty step".) At the same time, turn torso slightly to the left (9 o'clock), and raise right hand

43

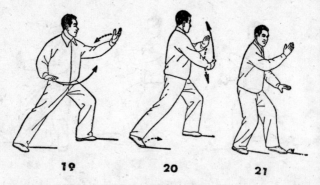

19   20   21

until it is in front of right temple, palm turned inward, while left hand moves downward until it stops in front of left hip, palm turned downward and fingers pointing forward. Look straight ahead. (Figs. 21-22)

Points to remember: Do not thrust chest forward. Arms should be rounded when they move up or down. Bend left leg slightly at knee. Shift of weight backward should be coordinated with the raising of right hand. Face 9 o'clock in the final position.

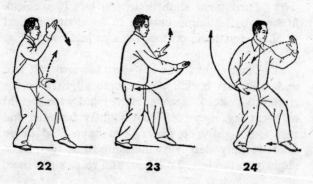

22   23   24

Series II

Form 4 Brush Knee and Twist Step on Both Sides

1) Turn torso slightly to the left (8 o'clock); right hand moves downward while left hand moves upward. Turn torso to the right (11 o'clock), right hand circles past abdomen and then upward to ear level with arm slightly bent and palm facing obliquely upward, while left hand moves first in an upward and then in a downward curve, stopping before right part of chest, palm facing obliquely downward. Look at right hand. (Figs. 23-25)

2) Turn torso to the left (9 o'clock). Left foot takes a step forward towards 8 o'clock to form a left "bow step". At the same time, right hand draws leftward past right ear and, following body turn, pushes forward at nose level with palm facing forward, while left hand drops and circles around left knee to stop beside left hip with palm facing downward. Look at fingers of right hand. (Figs. 26-27)

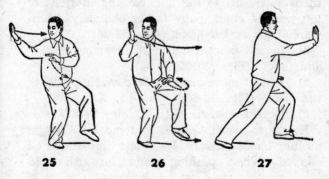

25   **26**   **27**

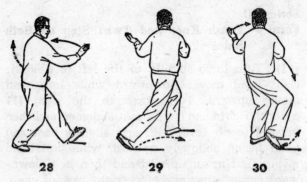

| 28 | 29 | 30 |

3) Sit back bending right knee slowly, shifting weight onto right leg. Raise toes of left foot and turn them slightly outward before placing foot flat on floor. Then bend the leg slowly. Turn body to the left (7 o'clock) and shift weight onto left leg. Bring right foot forward to the side of left foot and rest the toes on floor. At the same time, turn left palm up and, with elbow slightly bent, move left hand sideways and up to shoulder level, palm turning obliquely upward, while right hand, following body turn, makes an arc upward and then downward to the left, pausing in front of left part of chest, palm facing obliquely downward. Look at left hand. (Figs. 28-30)

4) Repeat movements in 2), reversing "right" and "left". (Figs. 31-32)

5) Repeat movements in 3), reversing "right" and "left". (Figs. 33-35)

6) Repeat movements in 2). (Figs. 36-37)

Points to remember: Keep torso erect while pushing hands forward. Waist and hips should be relaxed. When pushing palm forward, hold

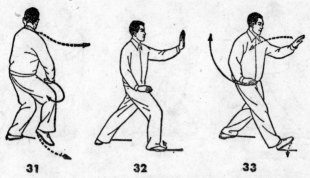

31 **32** **33**

shoulders and elbows down and keep waist relaxed. Movements of palm should be coordinated with those of waist and leg. Distance between heels should not be less than 30 cm. Face 9 o'clock in the final position.

Series II
Form 5   Hand Strums the Lute

Move right foot a half-step forward towards left heel. Sit back and turn torso slightly to the

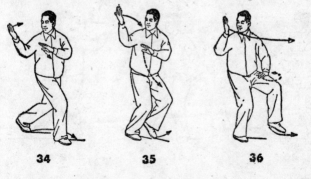

34 **35** **36**

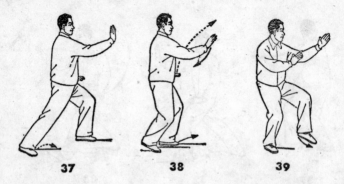

37   38   39

right (10-11 o'clock), shifting weight onto right leg. Raise left foot and place it slightly forward, heel coming down on floor and knee bent a little to form a left "empty step". Meanwhile, raise left hand in a curve to nose level, with palm facing towards the right and elbow slightly bent. Right hand moves downward until it reaches the inside of left elbow, palm facing to the left. Look at forefinger of left hand. (Figs. 38-40)

Points to remember: Body position should re-

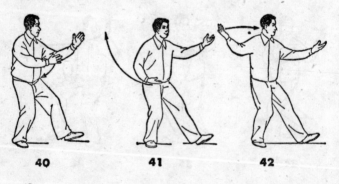

40   41   42

main steady and natural, chest relaxed and shoulders and elbows held down. Movement in raising left hand should be more or less circular. In moving right foot a half-step forward, place it slowly in position, toes coming down first. Weight transfer must be coordinated with the raising of left hand. Face 9 o'clock in the final position.

Series II
Form 6   Step Back and Whirl Arms on Both Sides

1) Turn torso slightly to the right (11-12 o'clock). Right hand makes a semicircle past abdomen and upward to shoulder level with palm facing upward and arm slightly bent. Turn left palm up and place toes of left foot on floor. First look to the right as body turns in that direction, then turn around to look ahead at left hand. (Figs. 41-42)

2) Bend right arm and draw hand past the ear before pushing it ahead with palm facing forward. Pull left hand back until it is beside waist, palm facing upward. At the same time, raise left

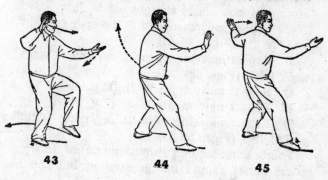

43   44   45

49

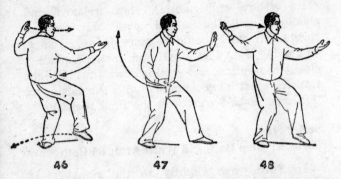

46   47   48

foot lightly and take a step backward towards 3-4 o'clock, placing it slowly on the floor toes first. Turn body to the left (8 o'clock) and shift weight onto left leg to form a right "empty step", with right foot pivoting on toes until foot points forward. Look at right hand. (Figs. 43-44)

3) Turn torso slightly to the left (6-7 o'clock). At the same time, carry left hand sideways and up to shoulder level, palm facing upward, while right palm is turned up. Eyes first look to the left as body turns in that direction, then turn around to look ahead at right hand. (Fig. 45)

4) Repeat movements in 2), reversing "right" and "left". (Figs. 46-47) .

5) Repeat movements in 3), reversing "right" and "left". (Figs. 48)

6) Repeat movements in 2). (Figs. 49-50)

7) Repeat movements in 3). (Fig. 51)

8) Repeat movements in 2), reversing "right" and "left". (Figs. 52-53)

Points to remember: In pushing out or drawing back, hands should not go straight but should

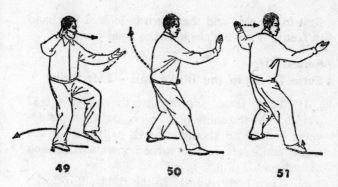

49   **50**   **51**

move in an arc. While pushing out hands, keep waist and hips relaxed. The turning of waist should be coordinated with hand movements. When stepping back, place toes down first and then slowly set the whole foot on floor. As body turns, pivot on toes of front foot until it comes in line with body. Move left leg slightly towards the left (or right leg slightly towards the right) when taking a step backward, taking care to prevent the feet from ending up in a straight line. Depending on the direction of body turn, look

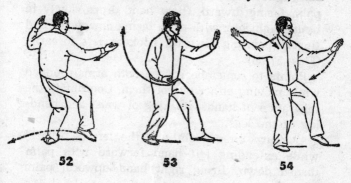

52   **53**   **54**

first to the side and then turn to look at the hand in front. Face 9 o'clock in the final position.

Series III
Form 7   Grasp the Bird's Tail — Left Style

1) Turn torso slightly to the right (11-12 o'clock). At the same time, carry right hand sideways and up to shoulder level, palm facing upward, while left palm is turned downward. Look at left hand. (Fig. 54)

2) Turn body slightly to the right (12 o'clock). Make a ball holding gesture in front of right part of chest, right hand on top. At the same time, shift weight onto right leg, draw left foot beside right foot and rest its toes on floor. Look at right hand. (Figs. 55-56)

3) Turn torso slightly to the left (11 o'clock). Left foot takes a step forward towards 8-9 o'clock. Turn torso a bit further to the left (10 o'clock), and bend left leg to form a "bow step", with right leg naturally straightened. Meanwhile, push out the rounded left forearm at shoulder level with palm facing inward. Right hand drops slowly to beside right hip, with palm facing downward and fingers pointing forward. Look at left forearm. (Figs. 57-58)

Points to remember: Keep both arms rounded while moving either one of them. Coordinate the separation of hands, relaxing of waist and bending of the legs.

4) Turn torso slightly to the left (9 o'clock) while extending left hand forward with palm turned down. Bring right hand upward, palm

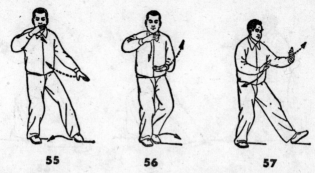

55   **56**   **57**

turning up, until it is below left forearm. Then
turn torso to the right (11 o'clock) while pulling
both hands down in such a way as to draw an
arc before abdomen, finishing with right hand extended sideways at shoulder level, palm up, and
left forearm lying across chest, palm turned inward.   At the same time, shift weight onto right
leg. Look at right hand. (Figs. 59-60)

Points to remember: While hands are pulled
down, do not lean forward or let buttocks protrude.   Arms should follow the turning of waist
and move in a circular path.

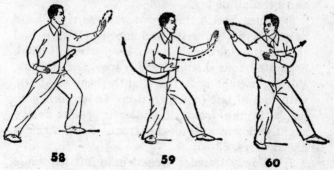

58   **59**   **60**

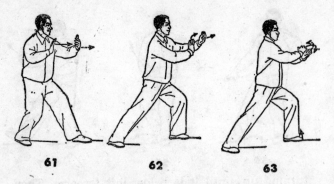

61   **62**   **63**

5) Turn torso slightly to the left (10 o'clock). Bend right arm and place right hand inside left wrist. Turn torso a little further to the left (9 o'clock). Press both hands slowly forward with right palm facing forward and left palm inward keeping left arm rounded. Meanwhile, shift weight slowly onto left leg to form a "bow step". Look at left wrist. (Figs. 61-62)

Points to remember: Keep torso erect when pressing hands forward; the movement of hands must be coordinated with the relaxing of waist and bending of leg.

6) Turn both palms downward as right hand passes over left wrist and moves forward and then to the right, ending on a level with left hand. Separate hands shoulder-width apart and sit back, shifting weight onto the slightly bent right leg, with toes of left foot turned up. Draw back both hands to the front of abdomen, palms facing slightly downward to the front. Look straight ahead. (Figs. 63-65)

7) Slowly transfer weight onto left leg while

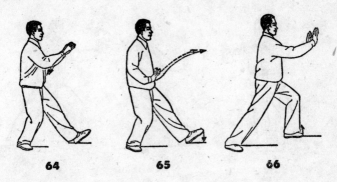

64   **65**   **66**

pushing hands forward and obliquely up with palms facing forward, until wrists are shoulder high. At the same time, bend left knee into a "bow step". Look forward. Face 9 o'clock in the final position. (Fig. 66)

Series III
Form 8   Grasp the Bird's Tail — Right Style

1) Sit back and turn torso to the right (12 o'clock), shifting weight onto right leg and turning toes of left foot inward. Right hand makes a

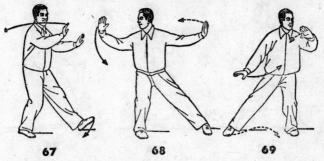

67   **68**   **69**

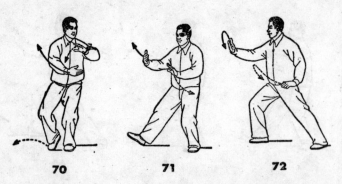

70　　　　**71**　　　　**72**

horizontal arc to the right, then moves downward past abdomen and upward to the left ribs, palm facing upward, forming a ball-holding gesture with left hand on top. Meanwhile, weight is shifted back onto left leg. Place right foot beside the left with heel raised. Look at left hand. (Figs. 67-70)

2) Repeat movements in 3) of Form 7, reversing "right" and "left". (Figs. 71-72)

3) Repeat movements in 4) of Form 7, reversing "right" and "left". (Figs. 73-74)

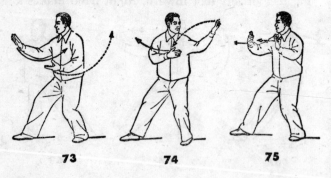

73　　　　**74**　　　　**75**

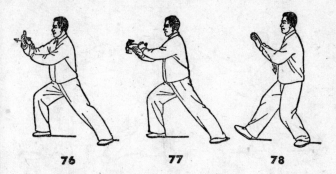

76 **77** **78**

4) Repeat movements in 5) of Form 7, reversing "right" and "left". (Figs. 75-76)

5) Repeat movements in 6) of Form 7, reversing "right" and "left". (Figs. 77-79)

6) Repeat movements in 7) of Form 7, reversing "right" and "left". (Fig. 80)

Points to remember: The same as those for Form 7. Face 3 o'clock in the final position.

Series IV
Form 9 Single Whip

1) Sit back and gradually shift weight onto

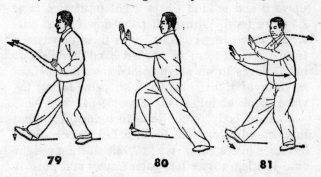

79 **80** **81**

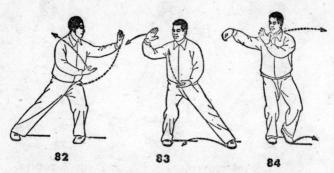

82   83   84

left leg while turning toes of right foot inward. Meanwhile, turn body to the left (11 o'clock). Move both hands leftward with left hand on top, until left arm is extended at shoulder level, palm facing outward, and right hand is in front of left ribs, palm facing obliquely inward. Look at left hand. (Figs. 81-82)

2) Turn body to the right (1 o'clock), shifting weight gradually onto right leg. Draw left foot next to the side of the right and rest its toes on floor. At the same time, right hand makes an arc upward and around to the right until arm is at shoulder level. With right palm now turned outward, bunch fingertips and turn them downward from wrist to form a "hooked hand", while left hand moves in an arc past abdomen and pauses in front of right shoulder with palm facing inward. Look at left hand. (Figs. 83-84)

3 Turn body to the left (10 o'clock) stepping forward with left foot towards 8-9 o'clock. Bend left knee into a "bow step". While shifting weight onto left leg, rotate left palm slowly and push it

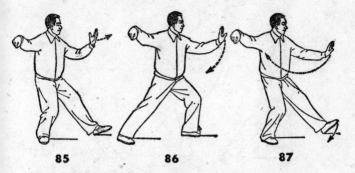

85   86   87

ahead with fingertips at eye level and elbow slightly bent. Look at left hand. (Figs. 85-86)

Points to remember: Keep torso erect and waist relaxed. Right elbow should be bent slightly downward and left elbow placed directly above left knee. Lower shoulders. Left palm turns as left hand is turned forward; do not turn it too quickly or abruptly. All transitional movements must be well coordinated. Face 8-9 o'clock in the final position.

Series IV
Form 10 Wave Hands Like Clouds — Left Style

1) Shift weight onto right leg and turn body gradually to the right (1-2 o'clock), while turning toes of left foot inward. Left hand makes an arc past abdomen and pauses in front of right shoulder with palm turned obliquely inward. At the same time, open right hand and turn palm outward. Look at left hand. (Figs. 87-89)

2) Turn torso gradually to the left (10-11 o'clock), shifting weight onto left leg. Left hand arcs past the face with palm turning slowly out-

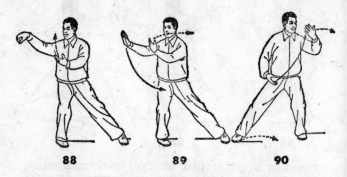

88   **89**   **90**

ward. Right hand makes an arc past abdomen and then upward to left shoulder with palm turned obliquely inward. Meanwhile, bring right foot parallel to the side of the left foot and about 10-20 cm. apart. Look at right hand. (Figs. 90-91)

3) Turn torso gradually to the right (1-2 o'clock), shifting weight onto right leg. Right hand continues to move to the right side past the face, palm turned outward, while left hand makes an arc past abdomen and upward to shoulder level with palm turned obliquely inward. Left foot then

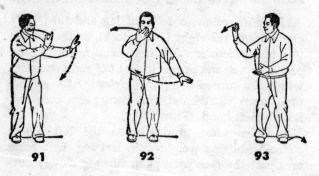

91   **92**   **93**

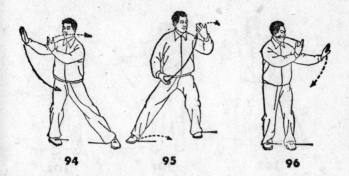

94   **95**   **96**

takes a side step. Look at left hand. (Figs. 92-94)

4) Repeat movements in 2). (Figs. 95-96)
5) Repeat movements in 3). (Figs. 97-99)
6) Repeat movements in 2). (Figs. 100-101)

Points to remember: Lumbar region of the spine serves as the axis for body turns. Keep waist and hips relaxed and avoid sudden rises or falls of body position. Arm movement should be natural and circular and should follow that of the waist. The pace must be slow and even. Maintain

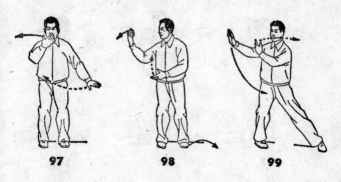

97   **98**   **99**

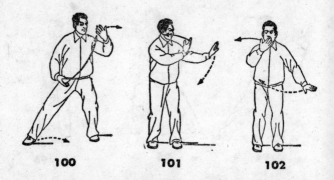

100   **101**   **102**

balance when moving lower limbs. Eyes should follow hands when they move past the face. Body in the final position faces 10-11 o'clock.

Series IV
Form 11   Single Whip

1) Turn torso to the right (1 o'clock). At the same time, right hand moves to the right and forms a hooked hand at a point slightly above shoulder level, while left hand makes an arc past

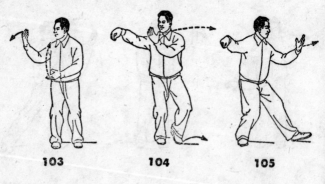

103   **104**   **105**

abdomen and then upward to right shoulder with palm turned inward. Weight is shifted onto right leg, while toes of left foot rest on floor. Look at left hand. (Figs. 102-104)

2) Movements are the same as in 3) of Form 9. (Figs. 105-106)

Points to remember: The same as those for Form 9. Face 8-9 o'clock in the final position.

Series V
Form 12   High Pat on Horse

1) Right foot takes a half-step forward; shift weight onto right leg. Open right hand and turn both palms upward with elbows slightly bent, while body turns slightly to the right (10-11 o'clock) with left heel gradually raised to form an "empty step". Look forward to the left. (Fig. 107)

2) Turn body slightly to the left (9 o'clock); draw right hand past right ear and push it forward with palm facing forward and fingers at

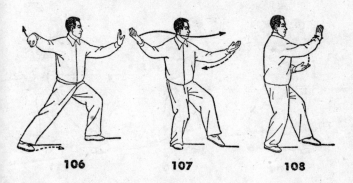

106   **107**   **108**

eye level pointing upward. Lower left hand until it comes in front of left hip, palm still facing upward. Meanwhile move left foot slightly forward with toes on floor. Look at right hand. (Fig. 108)

Points to remember: Hold torso erect and relaxed. Hold shoulders low and bend right elbow slightly downward. Do not let body rise or fall when shifting weight onto right leg. Face 9 o'clock in the final position.

Series V
Form 13   Kick with Right Heel

1) Cross hands by extending left hand, palm upward, onto the back of right wrist. Then separate hands and move in a downward arc with palms turned obliquely downward. Meanwhile, raise left foot and step forward towards 8 o'clock, forming a left "bow step" with toes turned slightly outward. Look straight forward. (Figs. 109-111)

2) Both hands move to outward in a circle and then down until they cross in front of chest, both

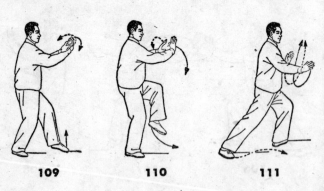

109   **110**   **111**

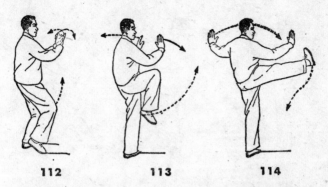

112   **113**   **114**

palms turned inward, with the back of left hand against the inside of right wrist. At the same time, bring right foot next to left foot and rest toes on floor. Look forward to the right. (Fig. 112)

3) Separate hands, extending them sideways at shoulder level, with elbows slightly bent and palms turned outward. At the same time, raise right leg, bent at knee, and thrust foot gently forward towards 10 o'clock. Look at right hand. (Figs. 113-114)

Points to remember: Keep your balance. Wrists are level with shoulders when hands are separated. Left leg is lightly bent when right foot kicks forward, and the force of the kick should be initiated from the heel, with upturned toes pointing slightly inward. The separation of hands should coordinate with the kick. Right arm is parallel with right leg. Face 9 o'clock in the final position.

Series V
Form 14   Strike Opponent's Ears with Both Fists

1) Pull back right foot and keep it suspended

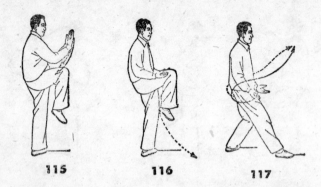

115   **116**   **117**

by bending knee so that thigh is level. Move left hand up and forward, then down next to right hand in front of chest, turning both palms up. Both hands make a circular movement downward, dropping to the sides of right knee. Look straight forward. (Figs. 115-116)

2) Right foot drops slowly to the floor at a point slightly to the right front of left foot, while weight is shifted onto right leg to form a "bow step". At the same time, drop both hands and gradually clench the fists. The hands then make an arc upward and forward from the sides to the front, coming together at ear level in a pincer movement, knuckles facing obliquely upward. Distance between fists is about 10-20 cm. Look at right fist. (Figs. 117-118)

Points to remember: Hold head and neck erect. Keep waist and hips relaxed and fists loosely clenched. Keep shoulders low and allow elbows to fall naturally with arms slightly bent. Face 10 o'clock in the final position.

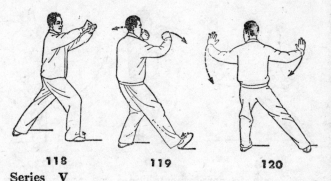

118 **119** **120**

Series V
Form 15 Turn and Kick with Left Heel

1) Bend left leg and sit back. Turn body to the left (6 o'clock) with toes of right foot pointing inward. Simultaneously open fists and separate hands in a circular movement extending them sideways slightly above shoulder level, palms facing forward. Look at left hand. (Figs. 119-120)

2) Weight is shifted onto right leg. Bring left foot to the side of the right and rest toes on floor. At the same time, circle both hands downward and to the sides and then inward and to the front until they cross in front of chest, with the back of right hand against the inside of left wrist, both palms facing inward. Look forward to the left. (Figs. 121-122)

3) Separate hands and extend them sideways at shoulder level, with elbows slightly bent and palms facing outward. Meanwhile, raise left leg with knee bent and then move foot gradually forward towards 4 o'clock. Look at left hand. (Figs. 123-124)

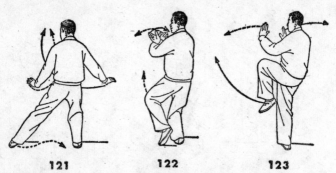

121   **122**   **123**

Points to remember: The same as those for Form 13, except that "right" and "left" are reversed. Face 4 o'clock in the final position.

Series VI
Form 16 Push Down and Stand on One Leg — Left Style

1) Pull back left foot and keep it suspended by bending knee so that thigh is level. Turn torso to the right (7 o'clock). Form a right hooked hand, while left palm is turned up and makes an arc up to the right until it comes in front of right shoulder and faces obliquely inward. Look at right hand. (Figs. 125-126)

2) Crouch slowly on right leg, stretching left leg sideways towards 2-3 o'clock. Left hand is extended sideways along the inner side of left leg, palm facing forward. Look at left hand. (Figs. 127-128)

Points to remember: When right leg is bent in a full crouch, turn toes of right foot slightly outward and straighten left leg with toes turned

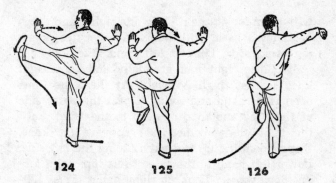

124　　　**125**　　　**126**

slightly inward; both soles are flat on floor.
Keep toes of left foot in line with heel of right
foot. Do not lean upper part of body too far forward.

3) Using heel as pivot, turn toes of left foot
slightly outward so that they come in line with
the outstretched leg; turn toes of right foot inward while right leg straightens and left leg
bends. Weight is thus shifted onto left leg.
Torso turns slightly to the left (4 o'clock) and
then rises slowly in a forward movement. At the
same time, left arm continues to extend forward,

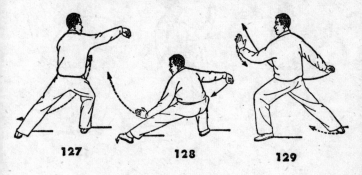

127　　　**128**　　　**129**

with palm facing the right, while right hand drops behind the back, with bunched fingertips pointing backward. Look at left hand. (Fig. 129)

4) Raise right foot gradually and bend right knee so that thigh is level. At the same time, open right hand and swing it past the outer side of right leg and then upward to the front, until the bent elbow comes just above right knee, fingers pointing up and palm facing the left side. Lower left hand to the side of left hip, palm facing downward. Look at right hand. (Figs. 130-131)

Points to remember: Keep torso upright. Bend the standing leg slightly. Toes should point naturally downward as right foot is raised. Face 3 o'clock in the final position.

Series VI
Form 17 Push Down and Stand on One Leg — Right Style

1) Place right foot down in front of the left and rest toes on floor. Turn body to the left (12

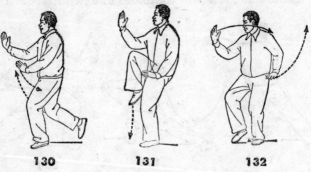

130   131   132

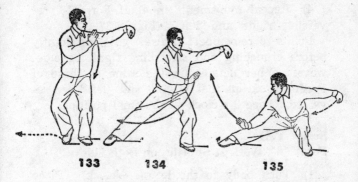

133   **134**   **135**

o'clock), using left toes as a pivot. At the same
time, left hand is raised sideways and upward
to shoulder level and is turned into a hooked
hand, while right hand, following the torso,
moves in an arc to the front of left shoulder with
fingers pointing up. Look at left hand. (Figs.
132-133)

2) Repeat movements in 2) of Form 16, reversing "right" and "left". (Figs. 134-135)

3) Repeat movements in 3) of Form 16, reversing "right" and "left". (Fig. 136)

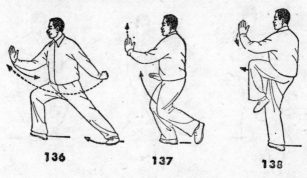

136   **137**   **138**

4) Repeat movements in 4) of Form 16, reversing "right" and "left". (Figs. 137-138)

Points to remember: Raise right foot slightly before crouching and stretching right leg sideways. Other details are the same as those of Form 16, except that "right" and "left" are reversed. Face 3 o'clock in the final position.

Series VII
Form 18   Work at Shuttles on Both Sides

1) Turn body to the left (1 o'clock). Place left foot on floor in front of right foot, with toes pointing outward. With right heel slightly raised, bend both knees to form a half "seat on crossed legs". At the same time, make a ball-holding gesture in front of left section of chest with the left hand on top. Then move right foot beside left foot and rest its toes on floor. Look at left forearm. (Figs. 139-141)

2) Body turns to the right (4 o'clock) and right foot steps forward to 4-5 o'clock to form

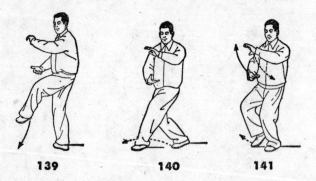

139   140   141

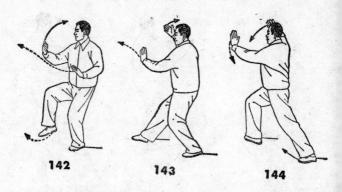

142   143   144

a "bow step". At the same time, right hand
moves upward, pausing just above right temple
with palm turned obliquely upward. Left hand
then moves downward to the left side and then
moves forward and upward to nose level, with
palm facing forward. Look at left hand. (Figs.
142-144)

3) Turn body slightly to the right (5 o'clock),
shifting weight slightly backward, with toes of
right foot turned outward a bit. Weight is then
shifted back onto right leg. Place left foot next
to right foot with toes on floor. Meanwhile,
make a ball-holding gesture in front of right section of chest with the right hand on top. Look
at right forearm. (Figs. 145-146)

4) Repeat movements in 2), reversing "right"
and "left". (Figs. 147-149)

Points to remember: Do not lean forward
when pushing hands forward, or shrug shoulders
when raising hands. Hand movements should
be coordinated with those of waist and legs.

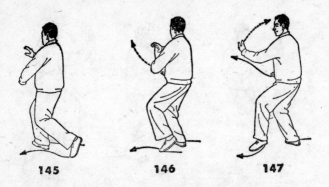

145   **146**   **147**

Distance between heels in "bow step" is about 30 cm. Face 2 o'clock in the final position.

Series VII
Form 19   Needle at Sea Bottom

1) Right foot takes a half-step forward. Weight is shifted onto right leg as left foot moves forward a bit with toes coming down on floor to form a left empty step. At the same time, turn body slightly to the right (3-4 o'clock). Lower

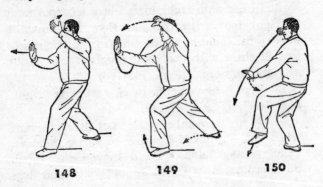

148   **149**   **150**

74

right hand in front of body, then raise it up beside right ear and, with body turning towards 2-3 o'clock, thrust it obliquely downward in front of body, with palm facing to the left and fingers pointing obliquely downward. Simultaneously, left hand makes an arc forward and downward to the side of left hip with palm facing downward and fingers pointing forward. Look at floor ahead. (Figs. 150-151)

Points to remember: First turn body slightly to the right and then to the left. Do not lean too far forward. Keep head erect and buttocks in. Left leg is slightly bent. Face 3 o'clock in the final position.

Series VII
Form 20 Flash the Arm

Turn body slightly to the right (4 o'clock). Step forward with left foot to form a "bow step". At the same time, raise right arm with elbow bent until the hand stops just above right temple.

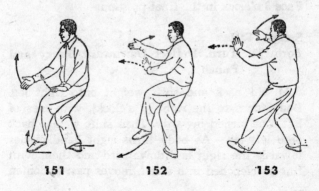

151   **152**   **153**

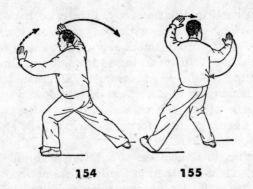

154   155

Turn palm obliquely upward with thumb pointing downward. Raise left hand slightly and push
it forward at nose level with palm facing forward. Look at left hand. (Figs. 152-154)

Points to remember: Hold torso in an erect
and natural position. Relax waist and hips. Do
not straighten left arm. Keep muscles of the
back relaxed. In pushing palm forward, the
movement should coordinate with the "bow step".
Distance between heels should not exceed 10 cm.
Face 3 o'clock in the final position.

Series VIII
**Form 21   Turn, Deflect Downward, Parry and
Punch**

1) Sit back and shift weight onto right leg.
Body turns to the right (6 o'clock), with toes of
left foot turned inward. Then shift weight back
onto left leg. As body turns right hand circles
towards the right and downward and then, with
fingers clenched into a fist, moves past abdomen

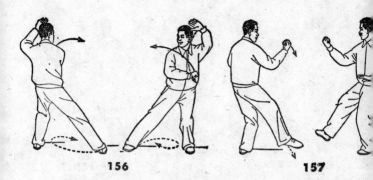

156 157

beside left ribs with knuckles up. At the same time, raise left arm above head with palm turned obliquely upward. Look forward. (Figs. 155-156)

2) Turn body to the right (8 o'clock). Right fist thrusts upward and forward in front of chest with knuckles turned down. Left hand lowers to the side of left hip with palm turned downward and fingers pointing forward. At the same time, draw back right foot and, without stopping or allowing it to touch floor, step forward with toes turned outward. Look at right fist. (Figs. 157-158)

3) Shift weight onto right leg and step forward with left foot. Meanwhile, parry with left hand moving up and forward from the left side in a circular movement, palm turned slightly downward, and pull right fist in a curve back to the side of right waist with knuckles turned downward. Look at left hand. (Figs. 159-160)

4) Left leg bends to form a "bow step". Meanwhile, right fist thrusts forward at chest level with the back of hand facing the right side.

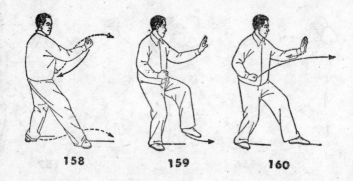

158 159 160

Pull left hand back to the side of right forearm. Look at right fist. (Fig. 161)

Points to remember: Clench right fist loosely. While pulling back the fist, forearm is first turned inward and then outward. While the fist strikes forward, right shoulder follows the movement and extends slightly forward. Hold shoulder and elbows down. Face 9 o'clock in the final position.

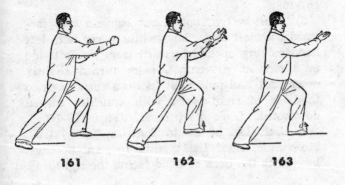

161 162 163

Series VIII
Form 22 Apparent Close-up

1) Left hand stretches forward from below right wrist; right fist opens. Turn palms up, separate hands and pull them back slowly. Sit back with toes of left foot raised, shifting weight onto right leg. Look forward. (Figs. 162-164)

2) Turning palms down in front of chest, push them downward past abdomen and then forward and upward. The movement finishes with wrists at shoulder level, palms facing forward. At the same time, bend left leg to form a "bow step". Look between the hands. (Figs. 165-167)

Points to remember: Do not lean backward when sitting back. Keep buttocks in. Relax shoulders and turn elbows slightly outward as arms are pulled back in unison with body movement. Do not pull arms back straight. The extended hands should be no farther than shoulder-width apart. Face 9 o'clock in the final position.

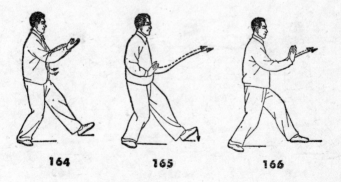

164   **165**   **166**

Series VIII
Form 23   Cross Hands

1) Bend right knee and sit back, shifting weight onto right leg. Body turns to the right (1 o'clock) as toes of left foot turn inward. Following body turn, both hands move to the sides in a circular movement at shoulder level, with palms facing forward and elbows slightly bent. Meanwhile, toes of right foot turn slightly outward and weight is shifted onto right leg to form a side "bow step". Look at right hand. (Figs. 168-169)

2) Weight is slowly shifted onto left leg and toes of right foot turn inward. Then bring right foot towards left foot so that they are parallel and shoulder-width apart; legs are gradually straightened. At the same time, move both hands down and cross them in front of abdomen, then raise the crossed hands to chest level with wrists at shoulder level, right hand on the out-

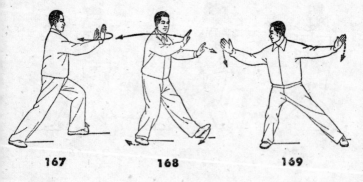

167   168   169

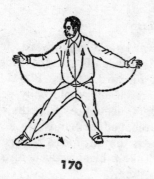

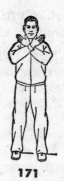

170

171

side and palms facing inward. Look straight forward. (Figs. 170-171)

Points to remember: Do not lean forward when separating or crossing hands. When taking the parallel stance, keep body naturally erect, with head held straight and chin tucked slightly inward. Keep arms rounded in a comfortable position, with shoulders and elbows held down. Face 12 o'clock in the final position.

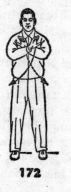

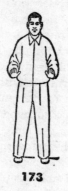

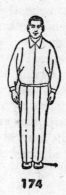

172

173

174

Series VIII
Form 24   Closing Form

Turn palms forward and downward while lowering both hands gradually to the side of hips. Look straight forward. (Figs. 172-174)

Points to remember: Keep whole body relaxed and slowly draw a deep breath (exhalation may be somewhat prolonged) as hands are lowered. Place left foot next to right foot after breathing becomes even. Take a brief walk before beginning any other activity.

Taijiquan: A Medical Assessment

Taijiquan as one of the methods of treatment prescribed in hospitals and sanatoriums has proved its efficacy in curing chronic diseases such as high blood pressure, neurasthenia and pulmonary tuberculosis. The salubrious effects of *taijiquan* are closely related to its characteristic features, namely: 1) the exercises require a high degree of concentration, with the mind free from distractions; 2) the movements are slow and uninterrupted; and 3) breathing is natural, sometimes involving abdominal respiration, and is performed in rhythmic harmony with body movements.

The high degree of concentration required in *taijiquan* exercises also benefits the function of the central nervous system. Training the mind and the body at the same time, these exercises stimulate the cerebral cortex, causing excitation in certain regions and protective inhibition in others. This enables the cerebrum to rest and relieves the cerebral cortex of the pathological excitation caused by ailments, thus helping to cure certain nervous and mental diseases.

The results of recently completed testing and examination involving *taijiquan* practitioners are given below. In this project, healthy subjects aged 50-89 were divided into two groups and given a battery of tests. Group A contained 32 persons who practised *taijiquan* regularly, while Group B (the control group) was composed of 56 individuals who did not engage in *taijiquan* training. In general, those in Group A were found to have stronger physiques characterized by more efficiently functioning cardiovascular, respiratory, osseous and metabolic systems.

Specific Findings

In regard to cardiovascular efficiency, the two groups underwent a functional test of stepping up and down a 40-cm-high bench 15 times within a minute. All but one person in Group A could bear this workload with normal responses in blood pressure and pulses. In the control group, however, the ability to bear this workload decreased and abnormal responses (such as type of step reaction and dystonia reaction) increased with the age of the subjects. The difference was also evident in electrocardiograms,* which sug-

---

* Abnormal patterns such as the prolongation of the P-R interval, the complex QRS and the QT duration, the reduction of the RV_5 amplitude, the depression of ST and the inverson of T, were found in 28.2 per cent of the subjects in Group A and 41.3 per cent in Group B.

gests that regular practice of *taijiquan* results in an increased supply of blood to the coronary arteries, more forceful heart contractions and improved hemodynamic function. Moreover, *taijiquan* may enhance the regulatory function of the central nervous system, improve the coordination of the internal organs, increase the tension of the vagus nerves, ensure adequate supplies of blood and oxygen to the tissues, and facilitate substance metabolism — all of which contribute to a lower rate of incidence of hypertension and arteriosclerosis. The average blood pressure was 134.1/80.8 mmHg. for Group A and 154.5/82.7 mmHg. for Group B, while the rate of incidence of arteriosclerosis was 39.5 and 46.4 per cent respectively.

Regular practice of *taijiquan* exercises can increase the elasticity of the lung tissues, the respiratory magnitude of the chest (which helps to retard the ossification of the rib cartilages) and the ventilatory capacity of the lungs, and improves the exchange of oxygen and carbon dioxide. The experiments showed Group A to be superior in both the respiratory discrepancy of the chest and vital capacity. Greater vital capacity results from a strong diaphragm and muscles of the thoracic walls, greater lung tissue elasticity and a lower rate of ossification of rib cartilages. For those whose breathing is already limited by ossification of rib cartilages, the abdominal respiration accompanying *taijiquan* exercises will improve ventilation of the lungs and, through rhythmic change of abdominal pressure, speed up blood flow and gas exchange in the alveoli pulmonum. This explains why, when completing the functional test, Group A subjects breathed more easily and recovered more quickly than those in the control group.

Taijiquan exercises can also strengthen bones, muscles and joints. Since many *taijiquan* movements hinge on the waist and involve a great deal of lumbar movement, systematic exercise can be beneficial to the form and structure of the lumbar vertebral and indeed the spinal column as a whole. Researchers noted that only 25.8 per cent of the subjects in Group A suffered from spinal column deformities, whereas in the control group the percentage was 47.2. Furthermore, fewer Group A subjects were victims of common, age-related hunchback deformities. Individuals in this group had more flexible spines, as evidenced by the fact that 77.4 per cent of them were able to touch their toes, as against 16.6 per cent in the control group. X-ray examination indicated that the rate of incidence of senile osteoporosis was 36.6 per cent for Group A and 63.8 per cent for Group B. Senile osteoporosis, which often leads to joint deformity and inflexibility, is a degenerative affliction mainly caused by inactivity of the osteoblasts. It may also be caused by such factors as reduced blood supply to the bones owing to arteriosclerosis and poor absorption of calcium and potassium from food due to the lack of hydrochloric acid in the gastric juices. Insofar as *taijiquan* can prevent or lessen such disorders, its role in retarding the aging process is noteworthy.

Limited data were obtained relative to the effects of *taijiquan* on substance metabolism. However, judging from the difference between the two groups in skeletal changes and in the incidence of arteriosclerosis, the beneficial effects of exercise appear significant, as far as the metabolism of fats, proteins and calcium and potassium salts is concerned. In recent years, several researchers in other countries have studied the role of physical exercises in delaying senescence. Cholesterol levels drop substantially for those who engage in regular exercise. Experiments conducted on elderly people with arteriosclerosis reveal that after five or six months' training, there is an increase of albumin and a marked decrease of globulin and cholesterol in the blood, while the symptoms of arteriosclerosis diminish markedly.

Conclusion

These findings, though preliminary and superficial, suggest that a regular programme of *taijiquan* exercises can be of benefit to one's physical well-being.

III. QIGONG

Qigong: Traditional Breath Energy Exercises

What is "*qigong*"?

The Chinese word *qi* literally means air or breath. In traditional Chinese medicine the meaning is broadened to refer to a person's vital energy (*yuan qi*), which includes, but is not limited to, the air one breathes in. *Qigong* is a series of breathing exercises aimed at stimulating vital energy so as to strengthen immunity to disease, adaptability to the external environment and the ability to repair internal damage. Traditional Chinese medicine holds that a person full of *yuan qi* will enjoy good health. Of course *qigong* is not a panacea; it must be practised in conjunction with other forms of exercise and therapy in order to effect a cure. To a great extent, all Chinese martial arts (*gongfu* or *kungfu*) rely on the mastery of *qigong* techniques for the attainment of mental and physical harmony.

All forms of *qigong* involve three mutually dependent basic processes: regulation of posture, regulation of respiration, and regulation of the mind.

Of the many *qigong* exercises, the following three forms are the most common: a) the relaxing exercise; b) the strengthening exercise; and c) the internal training exercise.

The Relaxing Exercise

This easily learned form has a wide range of applications.

Body position: Lie flat on back (Fig. 1), head on a pillow, arms laid comfortably by the sides, legs extended naturally, eyes and mouth slightly closed, teeth slightly clenched and tip of tongue touching hard palate.

Respiration: Breathe normally through nose — regularly, slowly, evenly and quietly. Say the word "calm" to yourself when inhaling and the word "relax" when exhaling. Relax a different part of the body at each respiration, first head, then arms, hands, chest, abdomen, back, small of the back, buttocks, legs and feet. After all the muscles are relaxed, concentrate on relaxing the blood vessels, nerves and viscera.

Frequency and duration of training: Individual fitness levels will be the primary determining factor. In general, a convalescent ordered to take a complete rest can perform this exercise three or four times a day, 20 to 30 minutes each time, while a person working part or full time can

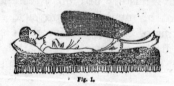

Fig. 1.

exercise once or twice a day, each time for 30 minutes. There is no definite length for a course of treatment. It usually takes two or three months, or even longer, to achieve noticeable effects.

The Strengthening Exercise

This form of exercise can be applied to cases of neurasthenia, hypertension, heart disease and pulmonary emphysema. The emphasis is on attaining a state of tranquillity rather than on respiration itself.

Body position:

a) Normal sitting position (Fig. 2): Sit erect on a square stool with feet flat on the ground, legs shoulder-width apart, knees bent at a 90 degree, thighs perpendiculer to trunk, palms resting in a relaxed manner on knees, elbows naturally bent, shoulders down, chin slightly withdrawn, chest in, and eyes, mouth and tongue as in the *Relaxing Exercise*.

b) Cross-legged sitting position (Fig. 3): Sit on a cushion, either with one leg folded over

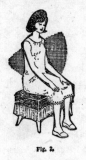

Fig. 2.

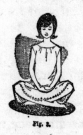

Fig. 3.

the other, or with both feet tucked under legs and both knees off the cushion. Buttocks should protrude slightly, head erect, back straight, shoulders down, chin slightly withdrawn and chest held in. Place hands below the navel or over the small of the abdomen, with thumbs locked and palms facing upward. For eyes, mouth and tongue follow the instructions in the *Relaxing Exercise*.

c) Standing position (Fig. 4): Stand with feet shoulder-width apart and slightly turned in, arms raised as if encircling a big tree, hands at shoulder level and elbows lowered, and fingers forming a circle as if clutching a large ball.

Respiration:

a) Natural breathing: Breathe through the nose as in the *Relaxing Exercise*.

b) Abdominal breathing: Inflate abdomen naturally while inhaling and deflate it while exhaling. With no pause between inspiration and expiration, breathing should gradually be deepened to reach six to eight full cycles per minute. This must be done naturally without forcing any deep breaths.

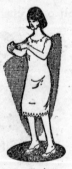

Fig. 4

Attainment of tranquillity: Focus your attention on abdomen — this is the basis of the *Strengthening Exercise*. In the initial stages of training, this may be achieved in the following ways:

— Count from one to ten as you breathe, one number for each

cycle of respiration. Start afresh if distractions cause your mind to wander. Repeat the one-to-ten count several times in succession.

— Clear your mind of all distracting thoughts and let it follow the rise and fall of your abdomen naturally while breathing.

— Direct your attention to a point about 5 cm. below the navel, allowing it to hover there without overstraining your mind. Begin again if your mind wanders.

The following progression is suggested for the *Strengthening Exercise*: (See page 92.)

The Internal Training Exercise

This is particularly suited for individuals suffering from duodenal ulcers, hepatitis, constipation and ptosis of the stomach. Stress is laid on breathing.

Body positions:

a) Normal sitting position (See the *Strengthening Exercise*);

b) Supine position (See the *Relaxing Exercise*);

c) Recumbent position (Fig. 5): Lie on your side (usually on the right) with head slightly forward, right arm bent and resting on pillow about 7 cm. away from head, palm upward, while

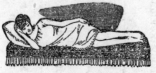

Fig. 5.

	Stage I (1st week)	Stage II (2nd-4th weeks)	Stage III (5th week and beyond)
Body position	Normal sitting position (or supine position for those in delicate health)	Normal or cross-legged sitting position	Sitting or standing position (the latter for stronger trainees)
Respiration	From natural to partial deep breathing	Natural deep breathing (abdominal)	
Attainment of tranquillity	Count respiration cycles or follow them mentally	Follow respiration cycles mentally or concentrate on a point 5 cm. below navel.	Concentrate on a point 5 cm. below navel
Frequency & duration	3-4 times daily, each time 15-20 min.	3-4 times daily, each time 30 min.	3-4 times daily, each time 30-45 min.
Requirements	1) Correct position 2) Regulated breathing 3) Freedom from distractions	1) Deep breathing down to diaphragm 2) Initial tranquillity 3) Training becomes habitual	1) Regular, deep, even breathing 2) Complete tranquillity 3) Noticeable benefits motivate further training

left arm is extended naturally, hand on hip with palm downward. Left leg rests on the right leg, both legs slightly bent.

Other positions may also be adopted provided they are natural and comfortable.

Respiration: Breathe abdominally through nose — inhale, exhale, pause (i.e. stop breathing) for 3-7 seconds, inhale, exhale, pause... repeat. During each pause, raise your tongue and meditate before dropping your tongue and inhaling again. Meditation consists in silently saying something meaningful to yourself such as "Be calm", "Relax" or "It's good to be calm and relax", each syllable lasting for one second. Progressively lengthen the pauses by saying more words. Do not exert yourself when holding your breath, nor hold it in your chest or throat. Simply stop breathing and focus your attention on the region of the navel.

The physiological function of the pauses requires further investigation, but preliminary studies suggest that these respiratory exercises bring about cyclic changes in internal abdominal pressure, which activate blood circulation in the abdomen and promote gastrointestinal peristalsis.

Attainment of tranquillity: Tranquillity is gradually acquired by coordinating respiration with the contemplation of selected words, which aids concentration and keeps the mind from wandering.

How Does *Qigong* Cure Diseases

Qigong has proved effective in treating certain

chronic disorders and, as indicated by recent experience in China, is particularly helpful to sufferers from stomach and duodenal ulcers, ptosis of the stomach, habitual constipation, neurasthenia and high blood pressure.

The role *qigong* plays is three-fold:

First, it helps restore vitality. By inducing a state of tranquillity, *qigong* allows the body to restore vital energy, build up disease-resistance and alleviate functional disorders. Physiological experiments show that when a person is in a tranquil state induced by *qigong* exercise, his cerebral cortex is in an inhibited state, which allays the over-excitation of cortical cells that may result in functional disorders. This may explain why *qigong* has proved beneficial in the treatment of neurasthenia, hypertension and gastric ulcers, which are all closely connected with the nervous system.

Secondly, it helps conserve energy. Experimental findings indicate that, in the course of performing *qigong* exercises, oxygen consumption is reduced by 30.7 per cent and energy metabolism by 20 per cent.

Thirdly, it massages the abdomenal cavity. *Qigong*, particularly the *Internal Training Exercise*, produces a massaging effect on the abdominal cavity through the mechanical action of breathing, since the diaphragm moves up and down over a much larger range than usual. Such massaging promotes gastrointestinal peristalsis, reduces the amount of extravasated blood in the abdomen and aids digestion and absorption. This is why one who practises *qigong* may have a sharpened appetite and put on weight — and also why *qigong* can cure habitual constipation and ptosis of the stomach.

How to Practise *Qigong*

To benefit from *qigong* exercises, the following principles should be observed:

1. Relax and remain at ease. First of all, relax your body. Don't shrug your shoulders or throw out your chest. Don't strain yourself to maintain your posture; always stay comfortable. All muscles must be relaxed, especially those of the lower abdomen. Clothes and belt should be loose. Second, set your mind at ease and adopt a cheerful attitude, free from all cares and worries. Regulate your breathing after initial relaxation is attained. It is usually during exhalation that you can feel yourself mentally and physically relaxed. Tranquillity is attained by focusing your attention on the exercise, banishing all other thoughts from your mind and avoiding as many external stimuli, such as sound and light, as possible. You will find yourself in a state of perfect calm wherein you will be unconscious of your own body weight. You may feel irritated at being unable to concentrate in the beginning. This is quite natural. Tell yourself to calm down and to be confident and patient. Persistent practice will bring steady progress.

2. Coordinate meditation with respiration. In *qigong* exercises, respiration must be guided by meditation. In other words, conscious efforts

must be made to regulate the rhythm of breathing, thereby directing the flow of vital energy to various parts of the body.

While the key to meditation lies in tranquillity, respiration cannot be considered satisfactory unless it is "fine, deep, long, slow, stable, leisurely and uniform". Both the *Strengthening Exercise* and *Relaxing Exercise* emphasize meditation while the *Internal Training Exercise* emphasizes respiration; but in any case, meditation and respiration must be coordinated.

3. Combine motion with stillness. As *qigong* calls for stillness and a minimum of motion, it should be supplemented with some active exercises for better therapeutic results. Active exercises should follow *qigong* exercises — in other words, motion after stillness.

4. Progress gradually. *Qigong* is an art that can be perfected only through long and disciplined practice. Start with the easier methods with regard to body position, breathing and the attainment of tranquillity. Each training period should last 15-20 minutes in the beginning and may be gradually lengthened as time goes on.

Here are some further suggestions:

1. About 15 minutes before practising *qigong*, stop reading and all other mental work, go to the toilet if necessary, and prepare yourself mentally for training.

2. Don't stand up abruptly after the exercise. Massage your face with both hands and rub your eyes gently before standing up slowly and stretching your limbs.

3. If you are short of breath or feel irritated while doing the exercises this may be due to inappropriate posture, incorrect breathing, a bad frame of mind or a lack of interest in exercising. Discover the cause and correct it.

4. If you feel dizzy or get a headache, this may be due to breathing with too much effort, impatience for quick results or a bad mood. Discover the cause and correct it.

5. Do not train on an empty or full stomach.

6. Suspend training when you are too tired or have a fever, diarrhea or a bad cold.

Prevention of Side Effects

Generally speaking, no side effects should be felt in the three forms of exercise provided they are performed properly. However, they may occur with beginners who are not used to the body positions and methods of breathing and meditation required in the exercises. These side effects can easily be prevented or overcome.

(A) Side effects in posture:

1. A stiff back after sitting for a long time. This is either because you are not accustomed to sitting that way or because of incorrect posture. To avoid this trouble, start with the supine position and gradually attempt the sitting position; or change to the supine position when you tire from sitting; or simply shorten the time of sitting.

2. Numbness in the legs while sitting in the cross-legged position. This may be prevented by limbering up your legs before sitting. If numb-

ness still occurs, massage your legs, change position, or stand up and move about a little and then sit down again.

(B) Side effects in respiration:

1. Difficulty in breathing and restlessness, usually caused by forced deep breathing. Take a short walk in the room and calm yourself before resuming the meditation.
2. Shortness of breath or a stitch in the side. This usually happens when you breathe too hard, try to hold your breath too long, or "trap" your breath in the chest or throat. Symptoms will disappear once these faults are overcome.

(C) Side effects in meditation:

1. Lethargy. In most cases, this occurs when lying down or due to mental exhaustion. You may feel better if you sit up or gaze at the tip of your nose with half-closed eyes. Don't practise *qigong* exercises when you are overtired. To prevent drowsiness, which is quite common with beginners, sip some hot tea and take a short walk before sitting down to meditate.
2. Extraordinary sensations. Sometimes, while in a state of deep tranquillity, you may feel numbness, itchiness, pins and needles or a burning sensation in the skin or muscles of some parts of your body. By concentrating your meditation on the small of the abdomen and refraining from breathing too deeply, these symptoms will soon disappear.

(D) Other side effects:

1. Palpitation of the heart. This usually occurs when, in a state of tranquillity, you breathe too deeply, hold your breath too long, or are too nervous. Discover the cause and correct it.

2. A throbbing sensation around the temples. Change your head position to relieve pressure on the ear.

Taiji Qigong

Taiji qigong is a simple series of exercises which combines the methods and benefits of *taijiquan* and *qigong*. Regular practice can contribute to relieving the symptoms of, and curing diseases of the digestive, respiratory and nervous systems, as well as heart disease, hypertension, rheumatism and arthritis.

I. Standing Form

Starting position:

Stand with the toes of both feet turned inward, the big toes one-sixth of a metre apart and heels one-third of a metre apart, with the main weight of the body resting on the balls of the feet. Keep both knees straight and upright, shoulders expanded and chest out; lower abdomen is drawn in and head inclined slightly forward. Concentrate the mind on *dantian* (a point about 4 centimetres below the navel). Close the eyes slightly, look at the tip of the nose and listen to your breathing.

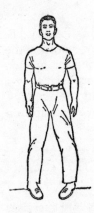

Movement 1.

Stand in the starting position, with hands hanging down naturally beside the legs. Breathe deeply from the abdomen, inhaling through the nose and exhaling through the mouth. Breathing should be slow, deep and even. Raise the tip of the tongue against the hard palate while inhaling, and let it relax while exhaling. The breaths should enter the lower abdomen. Silently count 15 respiration cycles (one inhalation and one exhalation for each cycle) before proceeding to the second movement.

Movement 2.

Extend both arms straight ahead at shoulder level, with the palms facing outward and fingers pointing upward.

Points to remember:

1) The thumb and fingers of both hands should be held close together.

2) Keep the mouth closed and raise the tip of the tongue against the hard palate.

3) Breathe in and out naturally through the nose. Breathing should be slow and even. Silently count 10 breaths before proceeding to the third movement.

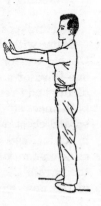

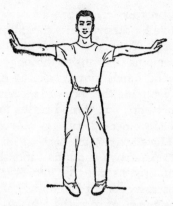

Movement 3.

Stand in the same starting position as before. Stretch the arms sideways at shoulder level to form a straight line, with the palms facing outward and fingers pointing upward. The points to remember are the same as in Movement 2. Again count 10 breaths before proceeding to the fourth movement.

Movement 4.

Stand in the same starting position as before. Extend both arms backward, palms facing downward and fingers held close together. Press the arms tightly against the ribs, with the chest inclined forward about 30 degrees. Raise both arms as high as possible without moving the body. The points to remember are the same as in Movement 2.

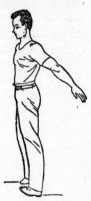

Count 15 breaths.

The above four movements should be performed continuously. The position of the toes (turned inward) remains unchanged throughout and only the arms and hands move. Take 50 breaths altogether to complete the series of movements. After every two weeks, add three breaths to Movement 1, two to Movement 2, two to Movement 3 and three to Movement 4, an increase of 10 breaths altogether. After two and a half months, the total number of breaths will be 100. Practice at this level of intensity for three months before increasing the number of breaths. In all cases, the increase should be gradual.

II. Sitting Form

Sit on bed. Stretch the legs straight, and keep the toes of both feet together and heels apart. Hold the stretched fingers close together, with the knuckles facing upward, and tuck the hands under the thighs. Hold chest out and draw in lower abdomen, with head inclined slightly forward. Concentrate the mind on *dantian*. Keep the mouth

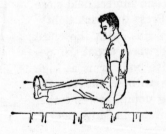

closed and press the tip of the tongue against the hard palate. Close the eyes slightly, look at the tip of the nose and listen to the breathing. Breathe naturally through the nose, with the breaths penetrating gradually into the lower abdomen. Silently count 100 breaths (or 50 if one is recuperating from an illness). Add 10 breaths every two weeks, so that the number of breaths increases gradually from 110 to 150, 160, and 200, depending on the condition of one's health. Be careful not to catch a cold in cold weather.

III. Lying Form

Lie on the back in bed. Stretch the legs straight, and keep the big toes about one-third of a metre apart and the heels slightly wider apart. Hold the stretched fingers close together, with the knuckles facing upward, and place the hands under the thighs. Rest the head on a pillow, with the shoulders naturally relaxed. Other movements are the same as in the sitting form. Silently count 100 breaths (50 at the beginning if one is recuperating from an illness). Follow the same rate of increase as in the sitting form. As one can usually practise longer while lying on one's back, the number of breaths can be increased to 300. Further increases will depend on the condition of one's health. In cold weather, cover the body with a blanket so as not to catch a cold.

IV. Walking Form

Place both hands behind the back, the left hand forming a relaxed fist which is held in the palm of the right hand. The forearms press gently against the upper part of the buttocks. Relax the shoulders and chest, and incline the head slightly forward. Walk slowly and in a relaxed manner, with the eyes and attention fixed on the toes, and the ears listening to the breathing. Breathing should be coordinated with the steps; the principle is to take the same number of steps for each exhalation as for each inhalation. The number of steps taken should increase gradually — from "two steps for each inhalation and two steps for each exhalation" to "nine steps for each inhalation and nine steps for exhalation". Take deep abdominal breaths, inhaling through the nose and exhaling through the mouth. It is advisable to do this exercise in the fields or woods where the air is fresh. Do it as if you are taking a stroll, and pay no attention to the time or distance.

V. Five Essential Points

In order to obtain the desired results, the following five points should be observed:

1) The mind should be at ease and remain tranquil.

2) The posture and movements should be correct.

3) Breathe slowly.

4) Increase the length of time for the exercise gradually.

5) Practise the exercise regularly every day.

VI. Points to Remember

1) The standing form is the most important

part of the exercise. The walking form can be done as a means of relaxation, after going through the movements in the sitting or lying position.

2) Do the exercise in a quiet place where the air is fresh, preferably where trees, flowers and other plants are growing.

3) It is preferable to do the standing exercise once after getting up in the morning and once before going to bed, and do the sitting exercise before taking a noon nap. The walking exercise should be done after the standing exercise. If there is not enough time, at least do the standing exercise once after getting up in the morning, or the sitting or lying exercise before getting out of bed.

4) In rainy, foggy or windy weather, do the exercise indoors.

5) Stop doing the exercise for some time if you have a cold or fever, or if you vomit blood.

6) Don't do the standing exercise less than half an hour after a meal; the sitting or lying exercise, however, can be done after a brief rest. The walking exercise can be done at any time.

7) Do not drink cold water immediately after the exercise. Take care not to catch a cold if you should start sweating.

8) Wear loose clothes when you do the exercise.

9) Do not talk with others when you do the exercise. If anyone should interrupt you, begin again.

10) Women who have reached the third month of pregnancy should stop doing the exercise.

VII. Reactions

At the beginning one may experience the following reactions:

1) Limbs ache.
2) Palms turn cold.
3) Arms shiver.
4) Chest and knees feel distended.

Don't worry about these reactions, since they are quite normal. Continue doing the exercise and they will disappear in a few days. After some time, however, one may experience other reactions such as flatulence, hiccuping, perspiration, or fever. These are good symptoms. After three or four months, your saliva will increase when you do the exercise and you will sense a slightly sweet taste in your mouth. In half a year you will feel extremely comfortable after exercises; but if you stop, you will feel rather uncomfortable.

Qigong Therapy: Simple Methods

1. Deep Breathing Exercise for Health Promotion

Before exercising, sit down quietly for a few minutes and clear your mind of all thoughts. Then close your eyes gently and mentally direct your attention to *dantian*, a point about 4 cm below your navel, while closing your mouth and inhaling through your nose slowly. Imagine drawing the breath down to *dantian* and holding it there for half a minute (which may be prolonged progressively to as much as two or three minutes). While holding your breath, pull in your navel as far as possible, holding this position for about one minute before releasing it. Exhale naturally without any conscious effort. Give no thought to your breathing and direct all your attention to *dantian*, imagining yourself "looking at" and "listening to" it throughout the exercise.

An initial practice session may last 20 minutes and be gradually lengthened to a maximum of 60 minutes. Walk around for 50 or 60 steps after each session. At least two sessions are required every day.

The exercise can be done in either sitting or supine position. It must be done on a daily basis without interruption to produce the desired effect. By the third month you will begin to feel warm and comfortable after doing the exercise. Years of regular practice will keep you fit and help extend your life.

2. Exercise for Curing Gastroptosis

Lie down on your back with your knees bent at about 115°, both feet lightly propped against the back of the bed, buttocks raised to a height of about 5 cm, arms naturally stretched, palms down, and with a pillow beneath your head (see diagram). Relax your whole body. Draw in a deep breath slowly and gently while placing your tongue on the hard palate. Then exhale slowly and release

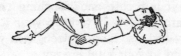

your tongue. Close your eyes and direct your attention to *dantian*.

The exercise should be done three or four times a day, each session lasting 30 to 60 minutes. Eat a proper diet of easily digestible food with more meals a day and less at each meal.

3. Ear Exercise for Curing Chronic Otitis Media

a) Clean your ears with cotton swabs before beginning.

b) You may either sit or stand when doing the exercise. In any case you must remain calm and relaxed. Put your palms over your ears and rub them in a circular movement 100 times. The rubbing should be forceful enough to produce a sensation of heat in your ears. Leave some space between the palm and the meatus lest the pressure of the palm should damage your ear.

c) With a rubbing motion of the palm, fold the auricle of each ear over the meatus and hold it there with the part of the palm near the base of the fingers. Then place the forefinger over the middle finger and snap it down on the mastoid bone behind the ear. Repeat this 100 times.

d) Do the exercise once every morning. Generally it will take effect in a week's time, but continued practice will increase the benefits.

4. Teeth Clenching Exercise

Holding your breath and clenching your teeth while urinating will help to keep your teeth firm and healthy and also help to strengthen your kidneys and add to your vital energy.

New Developments in *Qigong* Therapy

In recent years the curative properties of *qigong* have attracted increasing interest among medical personnel and patients of cancer and chronic diseases. Since the establishment of the Beijing *Qigong* Institute in December 1979, about a dozen coaching stations have been set up in parks and many more in factories and government organs. These stations have some 300 instructors teaching thousands of patients *qigong* exercises for preventative and curative purposes. According to an investigation made by the Institute, out of a total of 3,100 patients with chronic diseases who have practised *qigong* for 3-5 years, 25% have recovered completely, 44% have improved remarkably and 22% have improved slightly, while the remaining 9% have made no progress.

One of Beijing's most well known *qigong* masters is Guo Lin, who learned the art from her grandfather, a famous *qigong* master. After developing cancer of the uterus at the age of forty, Guo found herself too weak to do conventional *qigong* exercises and so worked out a new routine for her own use. She has continued to practise *qigong* for over twenty years and her cancer has never recurred.

Guo Lin has summarized her intensive studies of *qigong* theories and her own therapeutical experience in her book *Qigong: A New Method for Combating Cancer*, the first treatise ever written on this subject in China. Since 1973, she has given many lectures on *qigong* therapy and developed four courses: primary, secondary and advanced classes for ordinary chronic diseases, and a class for cancer therapy. The exercises she teaches fall into three main categories:

1. Natural Walking Exercises: These involve slow steps and armswinging coordinated with breathing.

2. Stick-rolling Exercises: The patient holds a 30-cm-long stick of rue (Zanthoxylum bungeanum) in his hands, rolling it gently between his palms while squatting and turning his trunk to right and left. The movements are synchronized with respiration.

3. Utterance Exercises: The patient utters long-drawn-out sounds, such as "ah", "yi" and "hi", which vary according to the parts of the body affected by the tumor.

Although the benefits of *qigong* exercises in curing chronic diseases including cancer have been proved, no satisfactory explanation of the whole process has been put forward. From the viewpoint of traditional Chinese medicine, it is presumed that by doing Guo's "walking exercises" which combine physical and mental activities through movement, meditation and regulated breathing, a patient can summon up his "internal vital energy" to bring about a balance between the "positive and negative elements" in his body. This clears his internal organs of obstructions and promotes circulation, thereby aiding recovery.

Initial investigations indicate that those cancer

patients who practise the walking *qigong* exercises regularly develop a greater ability in their phagocytes to destroy cancer cells; at the same time they find it easier to withstand the side-effects of radio- and chemo-therapies.

Another fascinating new development of *qigong* is *waiqi* or "outflowing energy" which some *qigong* masters can release through their fingertips either as a form of therapy or as an anaesthetic. One such master is Ma Chun.

While waving or pushing his palms from a distance of about one foot from the patient's diseased part, Ma emits *waiqi* from *laogongxue*, an acupuncture point in the palm. The patient feels a current coursing through his body, a feeling of numbness, cold and heat similar to that felt when a needle is inserted into an acupuncture point.

One patient Ma Chun cured suffered from compression fracture of the lumbar vertebrae and had long been confined to his hospital bed. When Ma released his *waiqi* in the direction of the patient's waist from a distance of 40 cm, the patient felt a current of heat throughout his body, and there was sweat on the tip of his nose and a rhythmic beat in some of his muscles. After only 20 days of treatment, he was cured and left the hospital.

Since mid 1980, the Shanghai No. 8 People's Hospital has been using *waiqi* in some operations to partially or completely replace the use of anaesthetics. Of ten thyroidectomies performed in May and June of 1980 using *qigong* anaesthesia administered by Lin Housheng from the Shanghai Traditional Chinese Medicine Research Institute, the results of nine were rated "excellent" according to the standards set for acupuncture anaesthesia, and the tenth was classified "grade 3" because 10 ml of a local anaesthetic was used. Eight of the nine "excellent" operations were aided with the use of 50 mg of dolantin (the dosage permissible in acupuncture anaesthesia) while the ninth was performed without any drugs.

Using the *waiqi* released from his palm or fingers, Lin has developed various new treatment methods. One of these, called *qizhen* ("air needles"), consists of inserting a tiny needle into an acupuncture point and applying *waiqi* to the needle. Under the impact of *waiqi* the needle and the patient's muscles twitch as currents of heat penetrate into them.

Waiqi has been identified by Chinese nuclear scientists as a kind of low frequency modulated infrared radiation. A highly concentrated form of energy, it has been shown through clinical experiments to both kill cancer cells which are later discharged from the body, and to raise the degree of cancer immunity. Though its therapeutic effect in the treatment of cancer of the thyroid gland, esophagus, stomach and rectum has been ascertained, much still remains to be explored in this unique new branch of medicine.

IV. MASSAGE

Therapeutic Massage

Therapeutic massage in China has a very long history, and was described in *Huangdi Neijing (Yellow Emperor's Manual of Internal Medicine)*, the oldest extant medical treatise. There is a passage in the *Manual* which states that "if the body is benumbed as a result of the blocking of the *jingluo*,* it may be cured by massage". The names of ten volumes of *The Yellow Emperor and Qi Bo's Treatises on Massage* were listed in *The History of the Han Dynasty* written by Ban Gu (32-92 A.D.) of the Eastern Han dynasty, by the time of the Sui and Tang dynasties (581-907), special massage departments were established in the imperial court and the subject was included in the medical curriculum.

Further development took place in subsequent dynasties. The influx of Western medicine after the Opium War (1840-1842) enriched Chinese medical science, but for a variety of reasons, tra-

---

* *Jingluo* (or meridians), according to traditional Chinese medicine, is the network of main and collateral pathways which link up the viscera and different parts of the body surface. It is believed that vital energy circulates through these pathways and that acupuncture points are distributed along their lengths.

ditional Chinese medicine, including massage, became the object of prejudice and misunderstanding.

With the founding of the People's Republic in 1949, traditional Chinese medicine gained a new lease on life and developed under the policy of combining Chinese and Western medicine. Massage therapy has also gained wide acceptance in clinical practice.

Exercises to Prevent Colds

Note: *Exercises are performed in time to multiples of a basic 8-beat count.*
Begin by marching in position for two 8-beat counts.

I. Rubbing Hands.

Starting position: Stand straight with arms at sides. Spread legs to shoulder width.

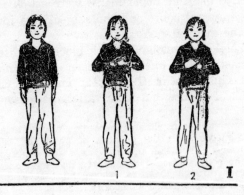

Movements:

1. Raise arms naturally in front of chest. With palms slightly curved inward, place left hand over right and rub hands around each other: First move left hand down towards you and right hand up away from you until right hand is over left hand.

2. Move left hand upward away from you and right hand downward towards you until left hand is over right hand again.

3, 5, 7, same as 1.

4, 6, 8, same as 2.

Repeat for 8 beats, returning to starting position on final beat.

II. Rubbing Face.

Starting position. Same as I.

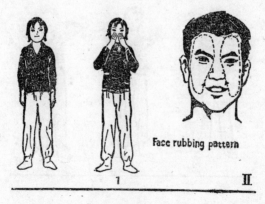

Face rubbing pattern

1   II.

Movements:

1. Pressing fingers of each hand together, bend elbows and place middle fingers on the sides of the nose. Move hands upward to hairline and continue outward and downward along hairline back up to starting point (see diagram).

Repeat same motion to two 8-beat counts, returning to starting position on final beat.

III. Rubbing Neck.

Starting position: Same as I.
Movements:

1. With fingers together, bend elbows upward and place hands on each side of the neck. Rub back and forth alternately for two 8-beat counts. Return to starting position on last beat.

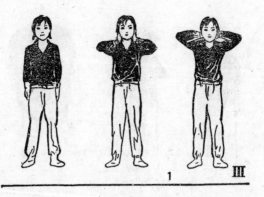

1   III

Requirement: The areas rubbed in the above three exercises should feel warm after rubbing.

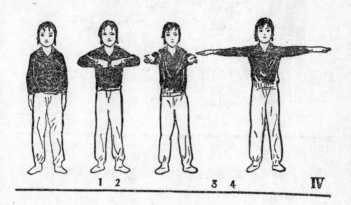

1 2   3 4   IV

IV. Chest-Expanding Exercise.

Starting position: Same as I.
Movements:

1. Make loose fists with palms facing downward. Bring arms horizontally in front of chest and stretch them vigorously to the side and back.

2. Repeat

3. Stretch arms horizontally in front of body with palms facing upward. Stretch arms vigorously to the side and back.

4. Repeat.

5 and 6, same as 1 and 2.

7 and 8, same as 3 and 4.

Repeat same motions to two 8-beat counts and return to starting position on final beat.

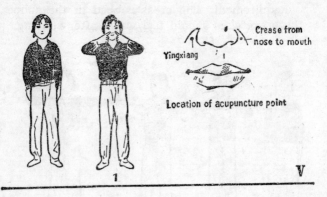

Yingxiang

Crease from nose to mouth

Location of acupuncture point

1

V

V. Massaging the *Yingxiang* Acupuncture Point

Starting position: Same as I.
Movements:

Make loose fists and press the *yingxiang* acupuncture point on both sides of nostrils (see diagram) with index fingers. Rotate fingers in circles on and around this point.

Repeat for two 8-beat counts. Return to starting point on final beat.

VI. Massaging the *Fengchi* Acupuncture Point

Starting position: Same as I.
Movements:

1. With fingers together, bend elbows and press *fengchi* acupuncture point on back of neck (see diagram) with index, middle and ring fingers. Rotate fingers in circles and around this point. Repeat for four 8-beat counts, returning to starting position on final beat.

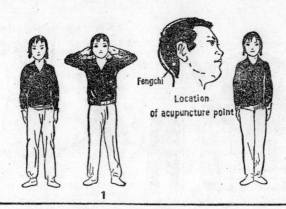

Fengchi

Location
of acupuncture point

1   VI

VII. Striking the *Zusanli** Acupuncture Point

Starting position: Stand at attention.

Movements:

1. Move left leg sideways to shoulder width. Raise arms overhead in a "V" position with palms forward. Look straight ahead and keep chest out.

2. Bend forward and touch ground with finger-tips.

3. Again touch ground with finger-tips.

4. Make fists. Strike the *zusanli* acupuncture point on left leg with inner side of left fist while swinging the right arm sideways.

5. Repeat movements with right leg and right fist.

6. Same as **4**.

7. Same as **5**.

8. Return to starting position.

---

* The *zusanli* acupuncture point is located about four fingers below knee-cap — see diagram.

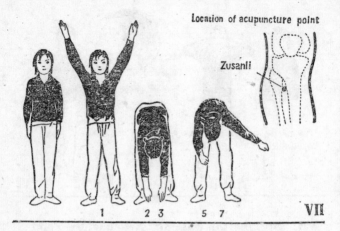

Location of acupuncture point

Zusanli

Repeat the above movements for four 8-beat counts.

VIII. Concluding Movements.

Starting position: Stand at attention.
Movements:

1. Make loose fists and raise arms to the side.

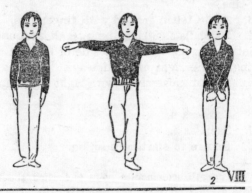

At the same time raise left thigh to 45 degree angle with the knee bent and shank relaxed.

2. Put down left leg and cross fists in front of the abdomen.

3. Same as 1, but raise right leg instead.

4. Same as 2.

Repeat for two 8-beat counts. In all movements, breathe evenly with muscles relaxed. Return to starting position on final beat.

Rubbing the Stomach

"Rubbing the Stomach" is a simple form of self-massage which has a particularly beneficial effect on the nervous and digestive systems. This particular set of exercises was developed from ancient and modern material on the subject in accordance with traditional and contemporary medical principles. Recent experiments have proved its efficacy in preventing and curing chronic diseases such as high blood pressure, neurasthenia, enterogastritis, constipation and gastric ulcer.

1. Posture

You may do the exercises in either sitting or lying position. In the sitting posture, hold your trunk upright, with the chest slightly drawn in, shoulders relaxed, eyes gazing ahead, feet flat on floor and shoulder-width apart, toes pointing forward. If you are on a bed, cross your legs comfortably. If you are ill or too weak to sit up, you may lie on your back with a pillow under your head, eyes gazing at the tip of your nose, legs together and slightly bent at knees, toes of both feet turned slightly outward and heels resting firmly on the bed.

2. Method

Before beginning, look at Illustration 1 to familiarize yourself with the acupuncture points and other parts of the body involved in the massage.

(1) Rubbing *zhongwan*: Place hands, one on top of the other, on the pit of your stomach. Using the pads of the index, middle and ring fingers (hereinafter referred to as the "middle three fingers") of both hands, exert light pressure in circular movement* around the *zhong-*

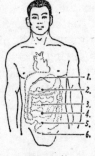 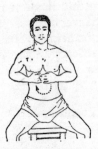

Illus. 1   Illus. 2

Illus. 1 Acupucture points and other vital parts of the body on which massages are applied.
1. xiphoid 2. *zhongwan* 3. navel 4. *qihai*
5. *guanyuan* 6. pubes

Illus. 2 Rubbing the stomach.

---

* The circular movement is used for all rubbing in this set of exercises.

wan point in a clockwise direction (Illus. 2). Do this 36 times.

(2) Rubbing the navel: Place hands one on top of the other as in (1). Starting from the left side of your navel, rub around it clockwise 18 times. Reversing the positions of the hands and starting from the right side of your navel, rub around it counterclockwise 18 times.

(3) Rubbing *qihai* and *guanyuan*: Place your hands one on top of the other as in (1). Starting from *qihai*, move clockwise down to *guanyuan* and up again to *qihai*. Do this 18 times. Then do the exercise another 18 times by reversing the position of the hands and rubbing in the counterclockwise direction.

(4) Stroking *renmai**: Place your hands one on top of the other as in (1). Starting from the pit of your stomach, stroke lightly down to the pubes, where the hands separate and, with the

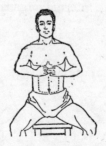

Illus. 3 Stroking *renmai*.

---

* According to traditional Chinese medicine, the *renmai* is a vein extending from the chin to the perineum.

middle three fingers of each hand, rub over the concavity of the ilium and up to the nipples, then back to the pit of the stomach where you place your hands one over the other again for the rubbing (Illus. 3). Repeat the whole process 36 times.

(5) Rubbing the whole stomach: Place left hand on left hip with thumb in front and fingers to the back. Rub with your right palm from the concavity of the right ilium, up to the upper right side of the stomach and crosswise to the upper left side, then down to the concavity of the left ilium before returning to the starting position (Illus. 4). Do the exercise 18 times with the right palm and another 18 times with the left.

(6) Stroking the waist: Place hands on waist with fingers drawn together and pointing forward and thumbs pressing below the lower ribs (Illus. 5). Press palms towards each other so that your belly protrudes a little, then release allowing belly to return to normal. Do this 18 times.

(7) Massaging internal organs: Sit with legs

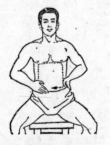

Illus. 4 Rubbing the whole stomach.

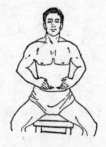

Illus. 5 Stroking the waist.

crossed comfortably, hands on your knees. Rotate trunk slowly nine times clockwise and another nine times in the counterclockwise direction (Illus. 6). The amplitude of rotation should be as large as possible.

8) Pressing: With one hand on hip (thumb in front and fingers on back), use the tips of the outstretched middle three fingers (the little finger and the thumb are bent) of the other hand for the manipulation. Slowly press hard on acupuncture points 5-7 times, each time releasing the pressure slowly. This method should not be used if you have calluses on your hands. Pressure points may be selected all over the abdomen, and should be spaced out about two and a half inches apart.

(9) Deep breathing: Take either the sitting or lying posture. If you sit, place hands on knees and fix eyes on the tip of your nose. If you lie supine, place hands at your sides. Before taking a deep breath, dispel all stray thoughts from your mind, ignore all noises, and concentrate your attention on *dantian*, a point about 4 centimetres

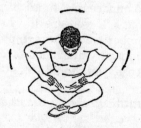

Illus. 6   Massaging internal organs.

below the navel. Relax completely and breathe naturally and quietly 20 times.

You may now proceed to deep breathing, which should be slow and even. Inhale through your nose while the tip of your tongue rests lightly on the hard palate, and exhale with your mouth as you release your tongue. Repeat 20-30 times. You should imagine an air current rising from *dantian* to your chest when you inhale, and returning to *dantian* as you exhale. Gradually deepen your breaths to increase ventilation. This will vary from person to person. Don't strain yourself or stop breathing at any moment. Towards the end of the exercise, you should gradually decrease the depth of breathing so as to recover your normal breathing pattern.

3. Points to Remember

(1) You can practise this set of exercises 2-3 times a day — morning, noon and evening, or you can do it in bed every morning and evening. The number of repetitions for each exercise is not restricted to what is specified in the foregoing sections; it may be increased to anywhere from dozens to hundreds of times as your physical condition permits. If you are ill, you should increase the number until the symptoms of your illness are temporarily alleviated or disappear entirely. In any case, you should feel good after each self-massage.

(2) Concentrate and breathe naturally throughout the exercises. Always let your mind follow your manipulations.

(3) Follow the principle of progression when learning the deep breathing exercise. Gradually increase the depth of your breathing and the number of repetitions.

(4) To achieve better results, you should rub on your bare skins rather than through your clothing. Keep your room warm to prevent yourself from catching a cold.

(5) The rubbing exercises should be done gently, slowly and continuously. Avoid applying excessive pressure that may injure your internal organs. This warrants special attention from women, especially older women, whose abdominal walls are thinner and more fragile than those of men. Women should also exert less pressure during menstrual periods.

(6) These rubbing exercises sometimes result in a quickening of gastrointestinal peristalsis, which in turn may lead to "stomach rumbling", flatulence, eructation, hunger pangs, or an urge for defecation. When you first practise deep breathing, you may feel a bit stuffy in your chest. These are all normal reactions and will disappear if you practise the exercises over a long period of time.

(7) Pregnant women are forbidden to do this set of exercises. So are people who suffer from malignant stomach tumours or from gastric or intestinal perforation, hemorrhage of internal organs or acute abdominal diseases. Don't do the exercises when you are hungry or have just eaten. If necessary, go to the bathroom before starting a session.

Massage Therapy for Meniere's Syndrome

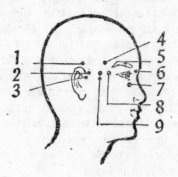

Illus. 1 Main acupuncture points for massage.

1. *qubin*   2. *shangguan*   3. *ermen*
4. *sizhukong*   5. *meiyao*   6. *yintang*
7. *chengqi*   8. *tongziliao*   9. *taiyang*

1. Study Illus. 1 to familiarize yourself with the acupuncture points to be massaged.

2. When you are not having an attack of Meniere's syndrome, you may massage the acupuncture points yourself in the order listed above. The "key points" *tongziliao, taiyang, shangguan* and *ermen* should be massaged half as many times again as the other points. Use either the index or middle finger to rub the "key points" and the *yintang* point, while using both fingers to rub the other points. Keep your eyes half shut and fists

half clenched while extending the forefingers and/or middle fingers to rub the points slowly in a clockwise direction (Illus. 2). Concentrate on the rubbing movements, which should be slow and just firm enough to produce the desired effect without causing discomfort. To conclude the exercise, use forefingers or middle fingers to stroke face lightly, starting from *tongziliao* and proceeding to *taiyang, shangguan* and *erman*. Repeat this several times. When you open your eyes, you will feel refreshed and comfortable.

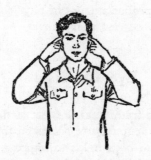

Illus. 2   Rubbing the *taiyang* points.

3.   When suffering from Meniere's syndrome, the same method may also be applied. In this case, first massage the "key points", especially *tongziliao* and *taiyang*. If you are too ill to manage it yourself, somebody else may do it for you, paying attention to rubbing the right points and applying the appropriate strength while rubbing.

To achieve better results, begin the massage at the first sign of illness. In more severe cases, take a sedative in the meantime.

Although the causes of Meniere's syndrome are still not known, it affects most people after mental or physical strain. It stands to reason, therefore, that positive results can be achieved by massaging the acupuncture points described above since such treatment stimulates blood circulation and can aid in relieving tension in the cerebrum. Still better results can be obtained if this method is supplemented by proper massage of the head, eyes and ears. As a preventive measure, one should take a proper amount of physical exercises and get sufficient rest every day.

Eye Exercises

According to traditional Chinese medicine, massaging certain acupuncture points on the face and the nape of the neck helps to improve the functioning of blood vessels and nerves and relieves strain on the eye muscles. A set of exercises based on this theory has been worked out and is widely practised among schoolchildren in China. Regular practice of these exercises has proved effective in improving eyesight and preventing or alleviating near-sightedness.

Exercise 1. Close eyes, place thumbs on the *jingming* points, squeeze and press towards the bridge of the nose (8 counts, 4 times).

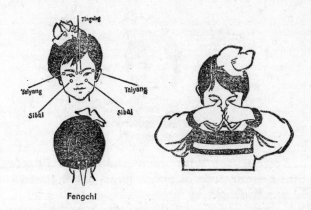

Fengchi

Exercise 2. Press *taiyang* points with thumbs and using the side of the second section of index fingers, massage the upper and lower parts of the sockets, beginning with the upper part (4 counts). Then massage the *taiyang* points with thumbs (4 counts). (Altogether 8 counts, 4 times.)

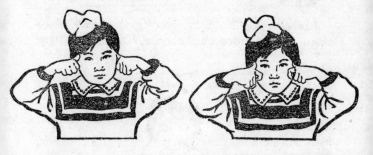

Exercise 3. Massage the *sibai* points directly below the sockets with index fingers (8 counts, 4 times).

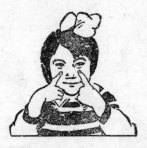

Exercise 4. With index and middle fingers massage the *fengchi* points (8 counts, 4 times).

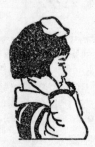 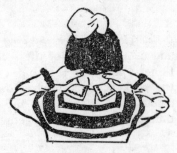

Exercise 5. Hold fingers together and place them on the sides of the nose. "Wash face" by

moving fingers up to the forehead, round the temples and down the cheeks (8 counts, 4 times).

Points to Remember:

1. Hands should be clean and fingernails clipped.

2. Do not do the exercises if there are boils or sores on the hands or face, nor if the eyes are injured or inflamed.

3. Concentrate when doing the exercises. Be sure you are massaging the correct points. The movements should be slow and gentle. Increase the pressure until you feel a bit sore.

4. It is better to do the exercises after reading or writing. Doing them once or twice every day will bring good results.

V. THE KEY TO LONGEVITY

Once upon a time a visitor at the seashore
Met ten centenarians still going strong.
In all sincerity he made a bow:
"Pray, how have you managed to live so long?"

Stroking his beard the first man replied,
"I've never touched liquor in all my life."

"I walk a hundred steps after each meal,"
The second greybeard rejoined with a smile.

Nodding in agreement, the third chimed in,
"I eat only vegetables and the simplest fare."

"I travel by foot instead of by wheel,"
Said the fourth, leaning on his cane.

The fifth added, flourishing the sleeves of his
robe,
"I do my laundry and all other chores with my
own hands."

Demonstrating a *taijiquan* form, the sixth ex-
plained,
"I do this fitness exercise every day."

Rubbing his nose the seventh observed,
"Keep the windows open and let the fresh air in."

The eighth, rosy-cheeked, remarked,
"I get a tan from the summer sun."

Twisting his moustache, the ninth stressed,
"Early to bed and early to rise."

The last gentleman concluded, raising his eye-
brows.
"I'm as merry as the day is long."

Always remember these old men's words,
For there's much truth in their song.
Do precisely as these men do,
If you want your days to be long.

图书在版编目(CIP)数据

中国传统的健身法:英文/《中国体育》杂志社编。
北京:新世界出版社,1995.12
ISBN 7－80005－310－5

I.中···
II.中···
III.健身运动－方法－中国－英文
IV.R161

中国传统的健身法

《中国体育》杂志社 编

*

新世界出版社出版
(北京百万庄大街 24 号)
北京大学印刷厂印刷
中国国际图书贸易总公司发行
(中国北京车公庄西路 35 号)
北京邮政信箱第 399 号 邮政编码 100044
1984 年(英文)第一版 1995 年第二次印刷
ISBN7－80005－310－5
01200
17－E－1745P